Secrets of Fat-Free Cooking

Over 150 fat-free and low-fat recipes from breakfast to dinner—appetizers to desserts

SANDRA WOODRUFF, RD

Avery Publishing Group
Garden City Park, New York

Text Illustrator: John Wincek
Interior Color Photographs: John Strange
Cover Photograph: John Strange
Cover Design: William Gonzalez
Typesetting: Bonnie Freid
In-House Editor: Joanne Abrams

Avery Publishing Group
120 Old Broadway
Garden City Park, NY 11040
1-800-548-5757

Cataloging-in-Publication Data

Woodruff, Sandra L.
    Secrets of fat-free cooking: over 150 fat-free & low-fat
recipes from breakfast to dinner—appetizers to desserts /
Sandra Woodruff.
        p. cm.
    Includes index.
    ISBN 0-89529-668-3

    1. Cookery. 2. Low-fat diet—Recipes. I. Title.

TX714.W66 1995   641.5'638
                                                  QBI94-21307

Printed in the United States of America

10 9 8 7 6 5 4

Contents

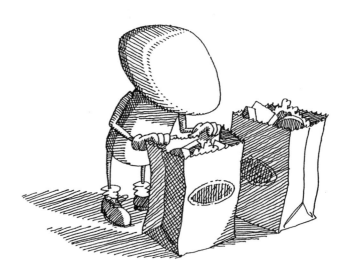

Acknowledgments

I would like to thank Rudy Shur, Ken Rajman, and Avery Publishing Group for providing me with the opportunity to publish this book. Special thanks go to my editor, Joanne Abrams, whose hard work and dedication have added so much to this book, and who, like everyone at Avery, is a pleasure to work with.

Thanks go to my dear friends and family members for their enduring support and encouragement. My sincere gratitude also goes to my clients and coworkers, whose questions and ideas keep me learning and experimenting with new things. Last, but not least, I would like to thank my significant other, Tom Maureau, and my faithful companion, Wiley, for always being there for me.

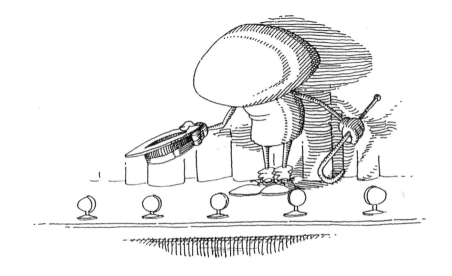

Preface

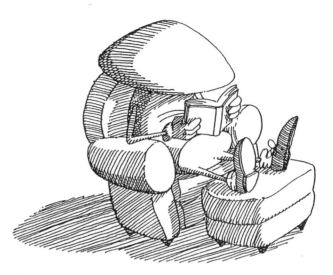

As a nutritionist, I have long been aware of the need to help people eliminate fat from their diet. I also know the importance of creating nutrient-rich dishes made with whole grains, fresh vegetables, and other ingredients that are as close as possible to their natural state. And because of my work as a teacher, I know that foods must be more than just healthy. They must be visually appealing and absolutely delicious, and they must be quick and easy to prepare. If they are not the former, people simply will not eat them. If they are not the latter, people simply will not make them.

Secrets of Fat-Free Cooking is the perfect book for people who want to reduce the fat in their diet, maximize their nutrition, and treat family and friends to delicious meals. From Golden French Toast, to Pot Roast With Sour Cream Gravy, to Hearty Oven Fries, to Refreshing Fruit Pie, every recipe has been designed to reduce fat and boost nutrition. Just as important, every recipe has been kitchen-tested to make sure that you enjoy success each and every time you make it, and people-tested to make sure that every dish you create is a hit.

Secrets of Fat-Free Cooking begins by explaining just why dietary fat should be reduced,

and just how much fat is allowable in a healthy diet. You will also learn about the many nonfat and low-fat ingredients that will help you reduce fat without reducing taste, and you will learn about the nutritional analysis that accompanies each and every recipe in this book.

Following this important information, each chapter focuses on a specific meal of the day or a specific type of dish. Looking for breakfast foods that are not only tempting enough to lure family members out of bed, but also nutritious enough to give them the energy they'll need until lunch time? Chapter 2, "Breakfasts for Champions," presents a wide selection of breakfast dishes, from Applesauce Pancakes to Zucchini Frittata. Or perhaps you want to serve fresh-baked breads, rolls, muffins, and biscuits that will add that special touch to family meals without wreaking havoc on your healthy lifestyle. "Bountiful Breads" will lead the way with a sumptuous selection of low- and no-fat homemade goodies that are as easy to prepare as they are delicious and nutritious. Still other chapters will show you how to make festive hot and cold hors d'oeuvres, like Chicken Fingers With Honey Mustard Sauce; warming soups, like Fresh Corn Chowder; refreshing salads, like Dillicious Potato Salad; wholesome vegetable side dishes, like Cranapple Acorn Squash; savory pasta dishes, like Bow Ties With Spicy Artichoke Sauce; hearty home-style entrées, like Simply Delicious Chicken and Dumplings; and meatless main dishes, like Eggplant Parmesan. And because for some of us, the meal just isn't complete until we've enjoyed dessert, there's a mouthwatering selection of cakes, cobblers, crisps, puddings, pies, cookies, and other treats designed to provide a sweet but nutritious conclusion to your fat-free meal.

It is my hope that *Secrets of Fat-Free Cooking* will prove to you, your family, and your friends, that any meal can be delicious and satisfying without being rich and fattening. So eat well and enjoy! As you will see, it is possible to do both—at every meal, and on every day of the year.

Introduction

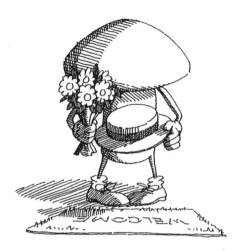

Making and eating great food is one of life's simplest yet greatest pleasures. And there is nothing wrong with enjoying good food—except that for too long, *good* often meant *greasy*. Butter, margarine, oil, mayonnaise, cheese, and other fatty ingredients were long considered essential for good cooking. We now know that all this fat—along with excess sugar and salt—has a tremendous impact on health. In fact, after smoking, diet is the number-one killer of Americans. Moreover, diet-related diseases like obesity, heart disease, cancer, and diabetes greatly affect the quality of life for millions of Americans.

The good news is that this awareness has led people to explore new ways of cooking and eating. As a result, many low-fat cookbooks are now available. But while these cookbooks do provide low-fat recipes, they often reduce fat and calories by using artificial fat substitutes and sweeteners, and they often rely on many highly refined, processed foods, as well. Because of these ingredients, nutrition is often compromised. *Secrets of Fat-Free Cooking* is a very different kind of cookbook. It was designed to help you create delicious low- and no-fat foods that are also high in nutrition.

As a nutritionist and teacher, I began looking for ways to reduce or totally eliminate the fat in

foods long before anyone heard the term "fat-free." Through years of experimentation and kitchen testing, I developed simple ways to do just this. But the recipes in this book are more than just low-fat. I have further improved the nutritional value of these recipes by using natural sweeteners like fruits and juices whenever possible to reduce the need for added sugar. Whole grains and whole grain flours have also been incorporated into these recipes for fiber and extra nutritional value. As an added bonus, the use of herbs, spices, and other seasonings, as well as minimal reliance on processed foods, has helped keep sodium under control.

Perhaps the best part of these recipes, though, is their simplicity. Every effort has been made to keep the number of ingredients, pots, pans, and utensils to a minimum. This will save you time and make cleanup a breeze—important considerations for most people today.

As you will see, watching your fat intake does not have to mean dieting and deprivation. This book is filled with easy-to-follow recipes for delicious dishes that your whole family will enjoy, as well as plenty of ideas for getting the fat out of your own favorite recipes. I wish you the best of luck and health with all your fat-free cooking!

1

1. Mastering Fat-Free Cooking

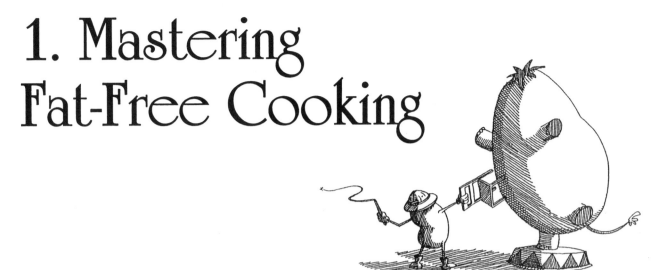

Who says you can't have your cake and eat it too? If you know the secrets of fat-free cooking, you can have just about anything you want—deceptively rich cheesecake, creamy fettuccine Alfredo, crispy Cajun chicken, cheese-filled lasagna, hearty Western omelettes, luscious quiches, and much more.

For too many years, eating healthfully has meant limited choices, deprivation, and extra hours spent shopping and cooking. "If it's good for you, it probably tastes awful," was the attitude that emerged. Fortunately, this is far from true. *Secrets of Fat-Free Cooking* introduces you to new fat-free cooking techniques, and shows you how to use the latest nonfat and low-fat products in all your meals. The result? Foods that are never bland or boring, that are simple to prepare, and that your whole family will love.

In these pages, you will find recipes for a wide variety of delicious low-fat and fat-free dishes. You will be delighted by "defatted" versions of old favorites, as well as tempting new creations that will let you eat the foods you love without guilt. Perhaps just as important, this book will show you that contrary to popular belief, changing over to a low-fat lifestyle does not have to be an ordeal. As you will see, the recipes in this book will save you not just fat and calories, but time and effort, too. Most of these recipes are very simple to prepare, even for beginners, and are designed to create as little mess as possible, saving you cleanup time.

This chapter will explain why dietary fat should be reduced, and will guide you in budgeting your daily fat intake. In addition, you will learn about the various healthful ingredients used throughout this book—ingredients that will enable you to prune fat from every meal of the day.

BIG FAT PROBLEMS

Excess fat may well be the number-one dietary problem in America. With more than twice the calories of carbohydrates or protein, fat is a concentrated source of calories. Compare a cup of butter or margarine (almost pure fat) with a cup of flour (almost pure carbohydrates). The butter has 1,600 calories, and the flour has 400 calories. It's easy to see where most of our calories come from.

Besides being high in calories, fat is also readily converted into body fat when eaten in excess.

Carbohydrate-rich foods eaten in excess are also stored as fat, but they must first be converted into fat—a process that burns up some of the carbohydrates. The bottom line is that a high-fat diet will cause 20 percent more weight gain than will a high-carbohydrate diet, even when the two diets contain the same number of calories. So a high-fat diet is a double-edged sword for the weight-conscious person. It is high in calories, and it is high in the kind of nutrient that is most readily stored as body fat.

But high-fat diets pose a threat to much more than our weight. When fatty diets lead to obesity, diseases like diabetes and high blood pressure can result. And specific types of fats present their own unique problems. For example, eating too much saturated fat—found in meat, butter, and other solid fats—raises blood cholesterol levels, setting the stage for heart disease. Polyunsaturated fat, once thought to be the solution to heart disease, can also be harmful when eaten in excess. A diet overly rich in vegetable oils like corn, sunflower, and safflower oil, as well as products made from these oils, can alter body chemistry to favor the development of blood clots, high blood pressure, and inflammatory diseases. Too much polyunsaturated fat can also promote free-radical damage to cells, contributing to heart disease and cancer.

Where do monounsaturated fats fit in? Monounsaturated fats—found in olive oil, canola oil, avocados, and nuts—have no known harmful effects other than being a concentrated source of calories, like all fats.

Considering the problems caused by excess fat, you may think it would be best to completely eliminate fat from your diet. But the fact is, we do need some dietary fat. For instance, linoleic acid, a polyunsaturated fat naturally abundant in nuts and seeds, is essential for life. The average adult needs a minimum of 3 to 6 grams of linoleic acid per day—the amount present in one to two teaspoonfuls of polyunsaturated vegetable oil, or one to two tablespoonfuls of nuts or seeds. Linolenic acid, a fat present mainly in fish and green plants, is also essential for good health. And some dietary fat is needed so that we may absorb fat-soluble nutrients like vitamin E.

Unfortunately, many people are getting too much of a good thing. The liberal use of foods like mayonnaise, oil-based salad dressings, margarine, and cooking oils has created an unhealthy overdose of linoleic acid in the American diet. And, of course, most people also eat far too much saturated fat. How can we correct this? We can minimize the use of refined vegetable oils and table fats, and eat a diet rich in whole grains, vegetables, and fruits, with moderate amounts of nuts and seeds, fish, and lean meats, if desired. This is what *Secrets of Fat-Free Cooking* is all about. In the remainder of this chapter, you will learn how to budget your daily fat intake, and you will become acquainted with the healthful foods that will help you prune the fat from your diet and maximize the nutrients. Throughout the rest of the book, you will learn how to use these foods to create delicious, healthful fare that you will be proud to serve, and your family will love to eat.

BUDGETING YOUR FAT

For most people, close to 40 percent of the calories in their diet come from fat. However, currently it is recommended that fat calories constitute no more than 30 percent of the diet, and, in fact, 20 to 25 percent would be even better in most cases. So the amount of fat you should eat every day is based on the number of calories you need. Because people's calorie needs depend on their weight, age, gender, activity level, and metabolic rate, these needs vary greatly among people. Most adults, though, must consume 13 to 15 calories per pound to maintain their weight. Of course, some people need even fewer calories, while very physically active people need more.

Once you have determined your calorie requirements, you can estimate a fat budget for yourself. Suppose you are a moderately active person who weighs 150 pounds. You will probably need about 15 calories per pound to maintain your weight, or about 2,250 per day. To limit your fat intake to 20 percent of your calorie intake, you can eat no more than 450 calories derived from fat per day (2,250 x .20 = 450). To convert this into grams of fat, divide by 9, as one gram of fat has 9 calories. Therefore, you should limit yourself to 50 grams of fat per day (450 ÷ 9 = 50).

The table at the bottom of this page shows two maximum daily fat gram budgets—one based on 20 percent of calorie intake, and one based on 25 percent of calorie intake. If you are overweight or underweight, go by the weight you would like to be. And keep in mind that although you have budgeted X amount of fat grams per day, you don't *have* to eat that amount of fat—you just have to avoid going over budget.

HOW LOW SHOULD YOU GO?

If you are like most people, you have discovered that for maximum health, you must reduce your daily fat intake. How low should you go? As discussed earlier, some fat is *necessary* for good health. Therefore, you should not try to consume less than 20 grams of fat per day. Of course, if you

eat a balanced diet rich in whole, natural foods, it would be almost impossible to eat less than this anyway. On the other hand, if you eat a diet rich in fat-free refined and processed foods, you could be at risk for a deficiency of essential fats, as well as deficiencies of other essential nutrients. This is why the recipes in this book so often use whole grains and other natural foods, and minimize the use of refined and processed foods.

Realize, too, that a very low-fat diet is not for everyone. If you have a specific medical problem, be sure to check with your physician or nutritionist before making any dramatic dietary changes.

ABOUT THE INGREDIENTS

Never before has it been so easy to eat healthfully. Nonfat and low-fat alternatives are available for just about any ingredient you can think of. This makes it possible to create a dazzling array of healthful and delicious foods, including low-fat versions of many of your favorite dishes. In the pages that follow, we will take a look at low-fat and nonfat cheeses, fat-free spreads and dressings, fat-free egg substitutes, ultra-lean meats, and many other ingredients that will insure success in all your fat-free cooking adventures.

Maximum Daily Fat Intakes

Weight	Recommended Daily Calorie Intake (13–15 calories per pound)	Fat Grams Allowed (20% of Calorie Intake)	Fat Grams Allowed (25% of Calorie Intake)
100	1,300–1,500	29–33	36–42
110	1,430–1,650	32–37	40–46
120	1,560–1,800	34–40	43–50
130	1,690–1,950	38–43	47–54
140	1,820–2,100	40–46	51–58
150	1,950–2,250	43–50	54–62
160	2,080–2,400	46–53	58–67
170	2,210–2,550	49–57	61–71
180	2,340–2,700	52–60	65–75
190	2,470–2,850	55–63	69–79
200	2,600–3,000	58–66	72–83

Low-Fat and Nonfat Cheeses

Americans have long had a love affair with cheese. For many years, though, people who wanted to reduce the fat in their diet had to also reduce the cheese, or even eliminate cheese entirely. Fortunately, a wide range of nonfat and low-fat products is now available, making it possible to have your cheese and eat it too. Let's learn about some of the cheeses that you will be using in your fat-free recipes.

Cottage Cheese. Although often thought of as a diet food, full-fat cottage cheese has 5 grams of fat per 4-ounce serving, making it far from diet fare. Instead, choose nonfat or low-fat cottage cheese. Puréed until smooth, these healthful products make a great base for dips and spreads, and add richness and body to casseroles, quiches, cheesecakes, and many other recipes. Select brands with 1 percent or less milk fat. Most brands of cottage cheese are quite high in sodium, with about 400 milligrams per half cup, so it is best to avoid adding salt whenever this cheese is a recipe ingredient. As an alternative, use unsalted cottage cheese, which is available in some stores.

Another option when buying cottage cheese is dry curd cottage cheese. This nonfat version is made without the "dressing" or creaming mixture. Minus the dressing, cottage cheese has a drier consistency; hence its name, "dry curd." Unlike most cottage cheese, dry curd is very low in sodium. Use dry curd cottage cheese as you would nonfat cottage cheese in casseroles, quiches, dips, spreads, salad dressings, and cheesecakes.

Cream Cheese. Regular full-fat cream cheese contains about 10 grams of fat per ounce, making this popular spread a real menace if you are trying to reduce dietary fat. A tasty alternative is light cream cheese, which has only 5 grams of fat per ounce. Another reduced-fat alternative is Neufchatel cheese, which contains 6 grams of fat per ounce. And, of course, nonfat cream cheese contains no fat at all. Like light cream cheese and Neufchatel, nonfat cream cheese may be used in dips, spreads, and sauces. Look for brands like Philly Free and Healthy Choice, and use the block-style cheese for best results.

When substituting nonfat cream cheese for full-fat cheese in cheesecakes, you may find that the texture of the cake is softer—more pudding-like—than that of traditional cheesecake. If this happens, try adding a tablespoon of flour to the batter for each cup of nonfat cream cheese used. This should produce a firm, nicely textured cake that is remarkably low in calories and fat.

Firm and Hard Cheeses. Both low-fat and nonfat cheeses of many types—including Swiss, Cheddar, Monterey jack, and mozzarella—are available in most grocery stores. Reduced-fat cheeses generally have 3 to 5 grams of fat per ounce, while nonfat cheeses contain no fat at all. Compare this with whole-milk varieties, which contain 9 to 10 grams of fat per ounce, and you will clearly see your savings in fat and calories.

Nonfat and reduced-fat firm and hard cheeses can be used in casseroles, in sauces—in any way that you might use their full-fat counterparts. Look for brands like Alpine Lace, Cracker Barrel Lite, Healthy Choice, Kraft Reduced-Fat, Kraft Healthy Favorites, Lifetime, Sargento Preferred Light, Jarlsberg Lite Swiss, and Weight Watchers.

Parmesan Cheese. Parmesan typically contains 8 grams of fat and 400 milligrams of sodium per ounce. Fortunately, reduced-fat and nonfat versions are available. A little bit of this flavorful cheese goes a long way, so even if you use regular Parmesan in any of the recipes in this book, the amount of fat per serving will be quite low.

Pasteurized Processed Cheese. Sold in blocks, in slices, and preshredded, this cheese is designed to melt smoothly, and so is intended as a cooking cheese for use in hot cheese dips, sauces, and similar dishes. When buying nonfat processed cheeses, look for brands like Healthy Choice, Lifetime, and Alpine Lace.

Ricotta Cheese. Ricotta is a mild, slightly sweet,

creamy cheese that may be used in dips, spreads, and traditional Italian dishes like lasagna. As the name implies, nonfat ricotta contains no fat at all. Low-fat and light ricotta, on the other hand, have 1 to 3 grams of fat per ounce, while whole-milk ricotta has 4 grams of fat per ounce.

Soft Curd Farmer Cheese. This soft, spreadable white cheese makes a good low-fat substitute for cream cheese. Brands made with skim milk have about 3 grams of fat per ounce, compared with cream cheese's 10 grams. Soft curd farmer cheese may be used in dips, spreads, and cheesecakes, and as a filling for blintzes. Some brands are made with whole milk, so read the label before you buy. Look for a brand like Friendship Farmer Cheese.

Yogurt Cheese. A good substitute for cream cheese in dips, spreads, and cheesecakes, yogurt cheese can be made at home with any brand of yogurt that does not contain gelatin. Simply place the yogurt in a funnel lined with cheesecloth or a coffee filter, and let it drain into a jar in the refrigerator for eight hours or overnight. When the yogurt is reduced by half, it is ready to use. The whey that collects in the jar may used in place of the liquid in bread and muffin recipes.

Nondairy Cheese Alternatives. If you choose to avoid dairy products because of a lactose intolerance or for another reason, you'll be glad to know that low-fat cheeses made from soymilk, almond milk, and Brazil nut milk are now available in a variety of flavors. Look for brands like Almondrella, Veganrella, and Tofurella.

Measuring Cheese

Throughout the recipes in this book, I have usually expressed the amount of cheese needed in cups. For instance, a recipe may call for one cup of cottage cheese or one-fourth cup of grated Parmesan. Since you will sometimes buy cheese in chunks and grate it in your own kitchen, or buy packages marked in ounces when the recipe calls

for cups, it is useful to understand that the conversion of cheese from ounces (weight) to cups (volume) varies, depending on the texture of the cheese. When using the recipes in *Secrets of Fat-Free Cooking,* the following table should help take the guesswork out of these conversions.

Cheese Equivalency Amounts

Cheese	Weight	Equivalent Volume
Cheddar	8 ounces	2 cups shredded or crumbled
Cottage Cheese	8 ounces	1 cup
Cream Cheese	8 ounces	1 cup
Farmer Cheese	8 ounces	1 cup
Mozzarella	8 ounces	2 cups shredded or crumbled
Parmesan	8 ounces	$2\frac{1}{4}$ cups grated
Ricotta	8 ounces	1 cup

Other Low-Fat and Nonfat Dairy Products

Of course, cheese isn't the only dairy product we use in our everyday cooking. How about the sour cream in dips, casseroles, and sauces, and the buttermilk in your favorite biscuits? Fortunately, there are low-fat and nonfat versions of these and other dairy products as well.

Buttermilk. Buttermilk adds a rich flavor and texture to baked goods like biscuits, muffins, and cakes, and lends a "cheesy" taste to sauces, cheesecakes, and casseroles. Originally a by-product of butter making, this product should perhaps be called "butterless" milk. Most brands of buttermilk contain from 0.5 to 2 percent fat by weight, but some brands contain as much as 3.5 percent fat. Choose brands that contain no more than 1 percent milk fat.

If you do not have buttermilk on hand, a good substitute can be made by mixing equal parts of nonfat yogurt and skim milk. Alternatively, place a tablespoon of vinegar or lemon juice in a one-cup measure, and fill the measure to the one-cup mark with skim milk. Let the mixture sit for five minutes, and use as you would nonfat buttermilk.

Evaporated Skim Milk. This ingredient can be substituted for cream in a variety of dishes. Use it to add creamy richness—but no fat—to quiches, sauces, cream soups, custards, and puddings.

Milk. Whole milk, the highest-fat milk available, is 3.5 percent fat by weight and has 8 grams of fat per cup. Instead, choose skim (nonfat) milk, which—with all but a trace of fat removed—has only about 0.5 gram of fat per cup. Another good choice is 1-percent milk, which, as the name implies, is 1 percent fat by weight and contains 2 grams of fat per cup.

Nonfat Dry Milk. Like evaporated skim milk, this product adds creamy richness, as well as important nutrients, to quiches, cream soups, sauces, custards, and puddings. One cup of skim milk mixed with one-third cup of nonfat dry milk powder can replace cream in most recipes. Or add this ingredient to fat-free cookies and brownies to enhance flavor and promote browning. For best results, always use *instant* dry milk powder, as this product will not clump.

Sour Cream. As calorie- and fat-conscious people know, full-fat sour cream can contain almost 500 calories and about 48 grams of fat per cup! Use nonfat sour cream, though, and you'll save 320 calories and 48 grams of fat. Made from cultured nonfat milk thickened with vegetable gums, this product beautifully replaces its fatty counterpart in dips, spreads, and sauces.

All brands of nonfat sour cream can substitute for the full-fat version in dips, dressings, and other cold dishes. However, some brands will separate when added to hot dishes like sauces and gravies. For these recipes, use a brand like Land O Lakes, which holds up well during cooking.

Yogurt. Yogurt adds creamy richness and flavor to sauces, baked goods, and casseroles. And, of course, it is a perfect base for many dips and

dressings. Like some brands of nonfat sour cream, however, yogurt will curdle if added to hot sauces or gravies. To prevent this, first let the yogurt warm to room temperature. Then stir one tablespoon of cornstarch or two tablespoons of unbleached flour into the yogurt for every cup of yogurt being used. You will then be able to add this tasty ingredient to your dish without fear of separation.

In your low-fat cooking, select brands of yogurt with 1 percent or less milk fat. If you must avoid dairy products, look for soy yogurt, which is available in health foods stores and many grocery stores.

Fat-Free Spreads and Dressings

Like cheeses, spreads and dressings were long a major source of fat and calories. Happily, many low-fat and nonfat alternatives to our high-fat favorites are now available. Let's learn a little more about these fat-saving products.

Margarine. If you are used to spreading foods with margarine, you can easily reduce your dietary fat by switching to a nonfat or reduced-fat margarine, and using it sparingly. Every tablespoon of nonfat margarine that you substitute for regular margarine will save you 11 grams of fat. You may be surprised to learn that you can also *bake* with reduced-fat margarine—and with light butter, too! Crisp cookies, light and tender cakes, biscuits, pie crusts, and other goodies can easily be prepared with half the fat by substituting reduced-fat margarine or butter for the full-fat products, and by making simple adjustments in the recipe. (For details on using these products in your baked goods, see the Low-Fat Cooking Tip on page 163.)

Mayonnaise. Nonfat mayonnaise is highly recommended over regular mayonnaise, which is almost pure fat. How can mayonnaise be made without all that oil? Manufacturers use more water and vegetable thickeners. Some commonly available nonfat brands are Kraft Free, Miracle Whip Free, and Smart Beat. Reduced-fat mayonnaise is also available, with half to two-thirds less fat and calories than regular mayonnaise. Look for brands like Hellmann's Reduced-Fat, Kraft Light, Miracle Whip Light, Blue Plate Light, and Weight Watchers.

Salad Dressings. Now made in a number of flavors, fat-free dressings contain either no oil or so little oil that they have less than 0.5 gram of fat per tablespoon. Use these dressings instead of oil-based versions to dress your favorite salads or as a delicious basting sauce for grilled foods.

Fat Substitutes for Baking

Almost any moist ingredient can replace the fat in cakes, muffins, quick breads, and other baked goods. The recipes in this book use a variety of fat substitutes. Most of these substitutes, including applesauce, fruit purée, fruit juice, nonfat buttermilk, yogurt, and mashed pumpkin, are readily available in grocery stores. Two additional substitutes—Prune Butter and Prune Purée—can be easily made at home using the recipes found in Chapter 11.

Egg Whites and Egg Substitutes

Everyone who cooks knows the value of eggs. Eggs are star ingredients in quiches, add lightness to casseroles, and are indispensable in a wide range of baked goods. Of course, eggs are also loaded with cholesterol. For this reason, the recipes in this book call for egg whites or fat-free egg substitute. Just how great are your savings in cholesterol and fat when whole eggs are replaced with one of these ingredients? One large egg contains 80 calories, 5 grams of fat, and 210 milligrams of cholesterol. The equivalent amount of egg white or fat-free egg substitute contains 20 to 30 calories, no fat, and no cholesterol. The benefits of these substitute ingredients are clear.

You may wonder why some of the recipes in this book call for egg whites while others call for egg substitute. In some cases, one ingredient does, in fact, work better than the other. For instance, egg substitute is the best choice when making quiches and puddings. In addition, because they have been pasteurized (heat treated), egg substitutes are safe to use uncooked in eggnogs and salad dressings. On the other hand, when recipes require whipped egg whites, egg substitutes do not work.

In most recipes, egg whites and egg substitutes can be used interchangeably. Yet, even in these recipes, one may sometimes be listed instead of the other due to ease of measuring. For example, while a cake made with three tablespoons of fat-free egg substitute would turn out just as well if made with three tablespoons of egg whites, this would require you to use *one and a half* large egg whites, making measuring something of a nuisance.

Whenever a recipe calls for egg whites, use large egg whites. When selecting an egg substitute, look for a fat-free brand like Egg Beaters. (Some egg substitutes contain vegetable oil.) When replacing egg whites with egg substitute, or whole eggs with egg whites or egg substitute, use the following guidelines:

1 large egg = 1½ large egg whites
1 large egg = 3 tablespoons egg substitute
1 large egg white = 2 tablespoons egg substitute

Ultra-Lean Poultry, Meat, and Vegetarian Alternatives

Because of the high fat and cholesterol contents of meats, many people have sharply reduced their consumption of meat, have limited themselves to white meat chicken or turkey, or have totally eliminated meat and poultry from their diets. The good news is that whether you are a sworn meat eater, someone who only occasionally eats meat dishes, or a confirmed vegetarian, plenty of lean meats, lean poultry, and excellent meat substitutes are now available.

The most important point to remember when including meat in meals is to keep portions to a modest 6 ounces or less per day. For perspective, a 3-ounce portion of meat is about the size of a deck of cards. Here are some suggestions for choosing the leanest possible poultry and meat.

Turkey

Although both chicken and turkey have less total fat and saturated fat than beef and pork, your very best bet when buying poultry is turkey. What's the difference between the fat and calorie contents of chicken and turkey? While 3 ounces of chicken breast without skin contain 139 calories and 3 grams of fat, the same amount of turkey breast without skin contains only 119 calories and 1 gram of fat.

Your best defense when preparing and eating poultry is removing the skin and any underlying visible fat. Doing just this eliminates over half the fat. Is there any advantage to removing the skin *before* cooking? A slight one. Poultry cooked without the skin has about 20 percent less fat than poultry that has the skin removed after cooking. And, of course, when the skin is removed after cooking, so is the seasoning. For this reason, the recipes in this book all begin with skinless pieces.

All of the leanest cuts of turkey come from the breast, so that all have the same amount of fat and calories per serving. Here is what you are likely to find at your local supermarket:

Turkey Cutlets. Turkey cutlets, which are slices of turkey breast, are usually about $\frac{1}{4}$-inch thick and weigh about 2 to 3 ounces each. These cutlets may be used as a delicious and ultra-lean alternative to boneless chicken breast, pork tenderloin slices, or veal.

Turkey Medallions. Sliced from turkey tenderloins, medallions are about 1 inch thick and weigh about 2 to 3 ounces each. Turkey medallions can be substituted for pork or veal medallions in any recipe.

Turkey Steaks. Cut from the turkey breast, these steaks are about $\frac{1}{2}$ to 1 inch in thickness. Turkey steaks may be baked, broiled, grilled, cut into stir-fry pieces or kabobs, or ground for burgers.

Turkey Tenderloins. Large sections of fresh turkey breast, tenderloins usually weight about 8 ounces each. Tenderloins may be sliced into cutlets, cut into stir-fry or kabob pieces, ground for burgers, or grilled or roasted as is.

Whole Turkey Breast. Perfect for people who love roast turkey but want only the breast meat, turkey breasts weigh 4 to 8 pounds each. These breasts may be roasted with or without stuffing.

Ground Turkey. Ground turkey is an excellent ingredient for use in meatballs, chili, burgers—in any dish that uses ground meat. When shopping for ground turkey, you'll find that different products have different percentages of fat. Ground turkey breast, which is only 1 percent fat by weight, is the leanest ground meat you can buy. Ground dark meat turkey made without the skin is 8 to 10 percent fat by weight. Brands with added skin and fat usually contain 15 percent fat. The moral is clear. Always check labels before making a purchase!

Chicken

Although not as low in fat as turkey, chicken is still lower in fat than most cuts of beef and pork, and therefore is a valuable ingredient in low-fat cooking. Beware, though: Many cuts of chicken, if eaten with the skin on, contain more fat than some cuts of beef and pork. For the least amount of fat, choose the chicken breast, and always remove the skin—preferably, before cooking.

Does ground chicken have a place in low-fat cooking? Like ground turkey, ground chicken often contains skin and fat. Most brands contain at least 15 percent fat, in fact, so read the labels carefully before you buy.

Beef and Pork

Although not as lean as turkey, beef and pork are both considerably leaner today than in decades past. Spurred by competition from the poultry industry, beef and pork producers have changed breeding and feeding practices to reduce the fat content of these products. In addition, butchers are now trimming away more of the fat from retail cuts of meat. The result? On average, grocery store cuts of beef are 27 percent leaner today than in the early 1980s, and retail cuts of pork are 43 percent leaner.

Choosing the Best Cuts and Grades. Of course, some cuts of beef and pork are leaner than others. Which are the smartest choices? The following table will guide you in selecting those cuts that are lowest in fat.

The Leanest Beef and Pork Cuts

Cut (3 ounces, cooked and trimmed)	Calories	Fat
Beef		
Eye of Round	143	4.2 grams
Top Round	153	4.2 grams
Round Tip	157	5.9 grams
Top Sirloin	165	6.1 grams
Pork		
Tenderloin	139	4.1 grams
Ham (95% lean)	112	4.3 grams
Boneless Sirloin Chops	164	5.7 grams
Boneless Loin Roast	165	6.1 grams
Boneless Loin Chops	173	6.6 grams

While identifying the lowest-fat cuts of meat is an important first step in healthy cooking, be aware that even lean cuts have varying amounts of fat because of differences in *grades*. In general, the higher and more expensive grades of meat, like USDA Prime and Choice, have more fat due to a higher degree of *marbling*—internal fat that cannot be trimmed away. USDA Select meats have the least amount of marbling, and therefore the lowest amount of fat. How important are these differences? A USDA Choice piece of meat may have 15 to 20 percent more fat than a USDA Select cut, and USDA Prime may have even more fat. Clearly, the difference is significant. So when choosing beef and pork for your table, by all means check the package for grade. Then look for the least amount of marbling in the cut you have chosen, and let appearance be your final guide.

Ground Beef. While ground turkey breast is the leanest ground meat you can find, low-fat ground beef is also available, giving you another option. One of your best bets is Healthy Choice ground beef. A mixture of lean beef and a small amount of oat flour, which is used to hold in moisture, this product is 4 percent fat by weight, giving it 33 calories and 1 gram of fat per ounce. Another good choice is 93-percent lean ground beef. Available in many grocery stores, this beef, as the label implies, is only 7 percent fat by weight.

If you are watching your sodium intake, you should be aware that some brands of low-fat beef, including Healthy Choice, contain salt. Before making your purchase, check the package's ingredients list and nutrition label. If salt is an ingredient, you will probably want to avoid adding more salt during cooking.

Lean Processed Meat

Because of our new fat-consciousness, low-fat sausage, ham, bacon, and lunch meats are now available, with just a fraction of the fat of regular processed meats. Many of these low-fat products are used in the recipes in this book. Here are some examples:

Sausage. Low-fat sausages are made either from turkey or from a combination of turkey, beef, and pork. These products contain a mere 30 to 40 calories and 0.75 to 3 grams of fat per ounce. Compare this with an ounce of full-fat pork sausage, which contains over 100 calories and almost 9 grams of fat, and your savings are clear.

When a recipe calls for smoked turkey sausage, try a brand like Healthy Choice, which has less than 1 gram of fat per ounce. When a recipe calls for ground turkey breakfast sausage, try a brand like Louis Rich. Many stores also make their own fresh turkey sausage, including turkey Italian sausage. When buying these fresh sausages, always check the package labels and choose the leanest mixture available.

Bacon. Turkey bacon, made with strips of light and dark turkey meat, looks and tastes much like pork bacon. But with 30 calories and 2 grams of fat per strip, turkey bacon has 50 percent less fat than crisp-cooked pork bacon, and shrinks much less during cooking. Besides being a healthier alternative to regular breakfast bacon, turkey bacon may be substituted for pork bacon in Southern-style vegetables, casseroles, and other dishes.

Lunch Meats. Many varieties of ultra-lean lunch meats are now available, including pastrami, corned beef, ham, and roast beef. These meats are ideal substitutes for fatty cold cuts in sandwiches and party platters. Keep in mind, though, that just like their full-fat counterparts, these meats are high in sodium, and so should be used in moderation.

Some processed meats are now labelled "fat-free." Since all meats naturally contain *some* fat, how can this be? The manufacturer first starts with a lean meat such as turkey breast, and then adds enough water—and usually extra salt and artificial flavors, as well—to dilute the fat to a point where the product contains less than 0.5 gram per serving. This means that part of your dollar actually pays for water, rather than meat. Fortunately, it is not necessary to go to this extreme when purchasing lean meats. Meats that are

labelled 96- to 99-percent lean—and therefore contain from 0.3 to 1 gram of fat per ounce—are lean enough to be included in a low-fat diet.

Vegetarian Alternatives

Nonmeat alternatives to ground meat can be substituted for ground beef or ground poultry in any of the recipes in this book. One good choice is Harvest Burger. Made from soybeans, Harvest Burger is rich in protein and has only about 1 gram of fat per ounce. Harvest Burger comes packaged as dry nuggets in individual pouches. When rehydrated, the contents of a single pouch is equivalent to one pound of ground meat. Harvest Burger can be shaped into meatballs or patties, and can replace ground meat in dishes like chili.

Texturized vegetable protein (TVP) is yet another alternative to ground meat. Made from defatted soy flour, TVP has about 0.3 gram of fat per ounce. Like Harvest Burger, TVP is packaged as dry nuggets that you rehydrate with water. TVP is an excellent ground meat substitute in chili, tacos, and many other dishes.

Fish and Other Seafood

Of the many kinds of fish that are available, some types are almost fat-free, while others are moderately fatty. However, the oil that fish provide contains an essential substance known as omega-3 fatty acids—a substance that most people do not eat in sufficient quantities. Omega-3 fatty acids are valuable because they can help reduce blood cholesterol, lower blood pressure, and prevent deadly blood clots from forming. This means that all kinds of fish, including the higher-fat varieties, are considered healthful.

Many fish are now raised on "farms." Do these fish offer the same health benefits as do fish caught in natural habitats? No. Farm-raised fish are fed grains, instead of a fish's natural diet of plankton and smaller fish. As a result, farm-raised fish contain as much or more fat than wild fish do, but are much lower in the beneficial omega-3 fatty acids.

What about the cholesterol content of shellfish? It may not be as high as you think it is. With the exception of shrimp, a 3-ounce serving of most shellfish contains about 60 milligrams of cholesterol, placing it well under the upper limit of 300 milligrams per day. An equivalent serving of shrimp has about 160 milligrams of cholesterol—just over half the recommended daily limit. Keep in mind, though, that all seafood, including shellfish, is very low in saturated fat, which has a greater cholesterol-raising effect than does cholesterol.

Fish is highly perishable, so it is important to know how to select a high-quality product. First, make sure that the fish is firm and springy to the touch. Second, buy fish only if it has a clean seaweed odor, rather than a "fishy" smell. Third, when purchasing whole fish, choose those fish whose gills are bright red in color, and whose eyes are clear and bulging, not sunken or cloudy. Finally, refrigerate fish as soon as you get it home, and be sure to cook it within forty-eight hours of purchase.

Grains and Flours

Just because a food is fat-free does not mean it is good for you. Fat-free products made from refined white flour and refined grains provide few nutrients, and can actually deplete nutrient stores if eaten in excess. Whole grains and whole grain flours, on the other hand, contain a multitude of nutrients such as vitamin E, zinc, magnesium, chromium, potassium, and many other nutrients that are lacking in refined grains. Whole grain products also add fiber to our diets, making our meals more satisfying. You see, fiber—like fat—provides a feeling of fullness. Fiber also helps maintain blood sugar levels, which helps keep hunger at bay. Adequate fiber is, in fact, an important part of a successful low-fat eating plan, as a diet of fat-free and low-fat refined foods is sure to leave you hungry.

Fortunately, once accustomed to the heartier taste and texture of whole grains, most people prefer them over tasteless refined grains. Following is a description of some whole grain products used in the recipes in this book. Many of these products are readily available in grocery stores, while others may be found in health foods stores and gourmet shops. If you are unable to locate a particular grain or flour in your area, it is probably available by mail order. (See the Resource List on page 177.)

Barley. This grain has a nutty light flavor, making it a great substitute for rice in pilafs, soups, casseroles, and other dishes. Hulled barley, like brown rice, cooks in about 50 minutes. Quick-cooking barley, which retains most of the fiber and nutrients of the long-cooking variety, can be prepared in only 10 to 12 minutes.

Barley Flour. Made from ground barley kernels, this flour is rich in cholesterol-lowering soluble fiber. Slightly sweet tasting, barley flour adds a cake-like texture to baked goods, and can be used interchangeably with oat flour in any recipe.

Bread Flour. Made from high-gluten wheat flour, this product is made especially for use in yeast breads. Bread flour also contains dough conditioners, such as ascorbic acid (vitamin C), that make doughs rise better.

Brown Rice. Brown rice is whole-kernel rice, meaning that all nutrients are intact. With a slightly chewy texture and a pleasant nutty flavor, brown rice makes excellent pilafs and stuffings.

Brown Rice Flour. Brown rice flour is simply finely ground brown rice. It has a texture similar to cornmeal, and adds a mildly sweet flavor to baked goods. Use it in cookies and waffles for a crisp and crunchy texture.

Buckwheat. Buckwheat is technically not a grain, but the edible fruit seed of a plant that is closely related to rhubarb. Roasted buckwheat kernels, commonly known as kasha, are available in most grocery stores, and make delicious pilafs and hot breakfast cereal.

Buckwheat Flour. Made from finely ground whole buckwheat kernels, buckwheat flour is delicious in pancakes, waffles, breads, and muffins.

Cornmeal. This grain adds a sweet flavor, a lovely golden color, and a crunchy texture to baked goods. Select whole grain (unbolted) cornmeal for the most nutrition. By contrast, bolted cornmeal is nearly whole grain, and degermed cornmeal is refined.

Millet. A staple in Oriental and African diets, this tiny round grain cooks in 15 to 20 minutes. Millet absorbs more water than most grains, and so is lower in calories. With a bland taste, millet is a good substitute for rice in almost any dish, and also makes an excellent hot cereal.

Oat Bran. Made of the outer part of the oat kernel, oat bran has a sweet, mild flavor, and is a concentrated source of cholesterol-lowering soluble fiber. Oat bran helps retain moisture in baked goods, making it a natural for fat-free baking. Look for it in the hot cereal section of your grocery store, and choose the softer, more finely ground products, like Quaker Oat Bran. Coarsely ground oat bran makes excellent hot cereal, but is not the best choice for baking.

Oat Flour. This mildly sweet flour is perfect for cakes, muffins, and other baked goods. Like oat bran, oat flour retains moisture in baked goods, reducing the need for fat. To add extra fiber and nutrients to your own recipes, replace up to one-third of the refined flour with an equal amount of oat flour. If you can't find oat flour in your local stores, you can easily make it at home by grinding quick-cooking rolled oats in a blender.

Oats. Loaded with cholesterol-lowering soluble fiber, oats add a chewy texture and sweet flavor

to muffins, quick breads, pancakes, cookies, and crumb toppings. They are also delicious in breakfast cereals and other dishes. Most of the recipes in this book use quick-cooking rolled oats. (Look for oats that cook in one minute.) Old-fashioned oats, which are cut slightly thicker, cook in 5 minutes.

Unbleached Flour. This is refined white flour that has not been subjected to a bleaching process. Unbleached white flour lacks significant amounts of nutrients compared with whole wheat flour, but does contain more vitamin E than bleached flour.

Wheat Bran. Unprocessed wheat bran—sometimes called miller's bran—is made from the outer portion of the whole wheat kernel. This grain product adds fiber and texture to breads, muffins, and other foods.

Whole Grain Wheat. Available in many forms, this grain is perhaps the easiest to use in the form of bulgur wheat. Cracked wheat that is pre-cooked and dried, bulgur wheat can be prepared in a matter of minutes and can be used to replace rice in any recipe.

Whole Wheat Flour. Made of ground whole grain wheat kernels, whole wheat flour includes the grain's nutrient-rich bran and germ. Nutritionally speaking, whole wheat flour is far superior to refined flour. Sadly, many people grew up eating refined baked goods, and find whole grain products too heavy for their taste. A good way to learn to enjoy whole grain flours is to use part whole wheat and part unbleached flour in recipes, and gradually increase the amount of whole wheat used over time. (One cup plus one tablespoon of unbleached flour can replace one cup of whole wheat flour in any recipe.)

When muffin, quick bread, cake, and cookie recipes call for whole wheat flour, **whole wheat pastry flour** works best, although regular whole wheat flour may be used with good results. Whole wheat pastry flour produces lighter, softer-textured baked goods than regular whole wheat flour because it is made from a softer (lower-protein) wheat and is more finely ground.

White whole wheat flour is another excellent option for baking. Made from hard white wheat instead of the hard red wheat used to make regular whole wheat flour, white whole wheat flour is sweeter and lighter tasting than its red wheat counterpart. To substitute white whole wheat flour for other flours, use the following guidelines:

---

1 cup white whole wheat flour =
1 cup unbleached (refined) wheat flour

---

1 cup + 1 tablespoon white whole wheat flour =
1 cup whole wheat pastry flour

---

1 cup + 1 tablespoon white whole wheat flour =
1 cup regular whole wheat flour

Sweeteners

Refined white sugar contains no nutrients. In fact, when eaten in excess, refined sugar can actually deplete body stores of essential nutrients like chromium and the B vitamins. Of course, a moderate amount of sugar is usually not a problem for people who eat an otherwise healthy diet. What is moderate? No more than 10 percent of your daily intake of calories should come from sugar. For an individual who needs 2,000 calories to maintain his or her weight, this amounts to an upper limit of 12.5 teaspoons (about $\frac{1}{4}$ cup) of sugar a day. Naturally, a diet that is lower in sugar is even better.

The baked goods and dessert recipes in this book contain 25 to 50 percent less sugar than traditional recipes do. Ingredients like fruit juices, fruit purées, and dried fruits; flavorings and spices like vanilla extract, nutmeg, and cinnamon; and mildly sweet oats and oat bran have often been used to reduce the need for sugar.

The recipes in this book call for moderate amounts of white sugar, brown sugar, and different liquid sweeteners. However, a large number of sweeteners are now available, and you should feel free to substitute one sweetener for another, using your own tastes, your desire for high-nutrient ingredients, and your pocketbook as a guide. (Some of the newer less-refined sweeteners are far more expensive than traditional sweeteners.) For best results, replace granular sweeteners with other granular sweeteners, and substitute liquid sweeteners for other liquid sweeteners. You can, of course, replace a liquid with granules, or vice versa, but adjustments in other recipe ingredients will have to be made. (For each cup of liquid sweetener substituted for a granulated sweetener, reduce the liquid by $\frac{1}{4}$ to $\frac{1}{3}$ cup.) Also be aware that each sweetener has its own unique flavor and its own degree of sweetness, making some sweeteners better suited to particular recipes.

Following is a description of some of the sweeteners commonly available in grocery stores, health foods stores, and gourmet shops. Those sweeteners that can't be found in local stores can usually be ordered by mail. (See the Resource List on page 177.)

Apple Butter. Sweet and thick, apple butter is made by cooking down apples with apple juice and spices. Many brands also contain added sugar, but some are sweetened only with juice. Use apple butter as you would honey to sweeten products in which a little spice will enhance flavor. Spice cakes, bran muffins, and oatmeal cookies are all delicious when made with apple butter.

Brown Rice Syrup. Commonly available in health foods stores, brown rice syrup is made by converting the starch in brown rice into sugar. This syrup is mildly sweet—about 30 to 60 percent as sweet as sugar, depending on the brand—and has a delicate malt flavor. Perhaps most important, brown rice syrup retains most of the nutrients found in the rice from which it was made. This sweetener is a good substitute for honey or other liquid sweeteners whenever you want to tone down the sweetness of a recipe.

Brown Sugar. This granulated sweetener is simply refined white sugar that has been coated with a thin film of molasses. Light brown sugar is lighter in color than regular brown sugar, but not lower in calories, as the name might imply. Because this sweetener contains some molasses, brown sugar has more calcium, iron, and potassium than white sugar. But like most sugars, brown sugar is no nutritional powerhouse. The advantage to using this sweetener instead of white sugar is that it is more flavorful and so can be used in smaller quantities.

Date Sugar. Made from ground dried dates, date sugar provides copper, magnesium, iron, and B vitamins. With a distinct date flavor, date sugar is delicious in breads, cakes, and muffins. Because it does not dissolve as readily as white sugar does, it is best to mix date sugar with the recipe's liquid ingredients and let it sit for a few minutes before proceeding with the recipe. Date sugar is less dense than white sugar, and so is only about two-thirds as sweet. However, date sugar is more flavorful, and so can often be substituted for white sugar on a cup-for-cup basis.

Fruit Juice Concentrates. Frozen juice concentrates add sweetness and flavor to baked goods while enhancing nutritional value. Use the concentrates as you would honey or other liquid sweeteners, but beware—too much will be overpowering. Always keep cans of frozen orange and apple juice concentrate in the freezer just for cooking and baking. Pineapple and tropical fruit blends also make good sweeteners, and white grape juice is ideal when you want a more neutral flavor.

Fruit Source. Made from white grape juice and brown rice, this sweetener has a rather neutral flavor and is about as sweet as white sugar. Fruit Source is available in both granular and liquid forms. Use the liquid as you would honey, and the granules as you would sugar. The granules do not dissolve as readily as sugar does, so mix Fruit Source with the recipe's liquid ingredients and let it sit for a few minutes before proceeding with the recipe.

Fruit Spreads, Jams, and Preserves. Available in a variety of flavors, these products make delicious sweeteners. For best flavor and nutrition, choose a brand made from fruits and fruit juice concentrate, with little or no added sugar, and select a flavor that is compatible with the baked goods you're making. Use as you would any liquid sweetener.

Honey. Contrary to popular belief, honey is not significantly more nutritious than sugar, but it does add a nice flavor to baked goods. It also adds moistness, reducing the need for fat. The sweetest of the liquid sweeteners, honey is generally 20 to 30 percent sweeter than sugar. Be sure to consider this when making substitutions.

Maple Sugar. Made from dehydrated maple syrup, granulated maple sugar adds a distinct maple flavor to baked goods. Powdered maple sugar is also available, and can be used to replace powdered white sugar in glazes.

Maple Syrup. The boiled-down sap of sugar maple trees, maple syrup adds delicious flavor to all baked goods, and also provides some potassium and other nutrients. Use it as you would honey or molasses.

Molasses. Light, or Barbados, molasses is pure sugar cane juice boiled down into a thick syrup. Light molasses provides some calcium, potassium, and iron, and is delicious in spice cakes, muffins, breads, and cookies. Blackstrap molasses is a by-product of the sugar-refining process. Very rich in calcium, potassium, and iron, it has a slightly bitter, strong flavor, and is half as sweet as refined sugar. Because of its distinctive taste, more than a few tablespoons in a recipe is overwhelming.

Sucanat. Granules of evaporated sugar cane juice, Sucanat tastes similar to brown sugar. This sweetener provides small amounts of potassium, chromium, calcium, iron, and vitamins A and C. Use it as you would any other granulated sugar.

Sugarcane Syrup. The process used to make sugarcane syrup is similar to that of making light molasses. Consequently, the syrup has a molasses-like flavor and is nutritionally comparable to the other sweetener.

Throughout our discussion of sweeteners, we have mentioned that some sweeteners are higher in nutrients than others. Just how much variation is there among sweeteners? The table at the bottom of this page compares the amounts of selected nutrients found in one-quarter cup of different sweeteners. Pay special attention to how the sweeteners compare with white sugar, the most refined of all the sweeteners.

Other Ingredients

Aside from the ingredients already discussed, a few more items may prove useful as you venture into fat-free cooking. Some ingredients may already be familiar to you, while others may become new additions to your pantry.

Barley Nugget Cereal. Whenever you want to replace or reduce the nuts in a recipe, try using a crunchy, nutty cereal like Grape-Nuts. The flavorful nuggets make a nice addition to crumb toppings, cookies, muffins, and other baked goods.

Couscous. A staple in African and Middle Eastern diets, couscous is actually pasta that has been shaped into small grain-sized pieces. Most of the couscous available in supermarkets is made from refined flour, but whole wheat couscous is also available, and is definitely a better nutritional bargain. Couscous cooks in less than five minutes, and is an excellent alternative to rice when used as a bed for stir-fries or in side dishes, salads, and casseroles.

Comparing Sweeteners

Sweetener (1/4 cup)	Calories	Calcium (mg)	Iron (mg)	Potassium (mg)
Apple Butter	130	10	0.5	176
Brown Rice Syrup	256	3	0.1	140
Brown Sugar	205	47	1.2	189
Date Sugar	88	10	0.4	209
Fruit Juice Concentrate (apple)	116	14	0.6	315
Fruit Juice Concentrate (orange)	113	23	0.3	479
Fruit Preserves	216	8	0	12
Fruit Source (granules)	192	16	0.4	142
Fruit Source (syrup)	176	15	0.4	138
Honey	240	0	0.5	27
Maple Sugar	176	45	0.8	137
Maple Syrup	202	83	1.0	141
Molasses, Blackstrap	170	548	20.2	2,342
Molasses, Light	172	132	4.3	732
Sucanat	144	41	1.6	162
Sugar Cane Syrup	210	48	2.9	340
White Sugar	192	1	0	2

Dried Fruits. A wide variety of dried fruits are available. Dried pineapple, apricots, prunes, dates, and peaches are available in most grocery stores, while health foods stores and gourmet shops often carry dried mangoes, papaya, cherries, blueberries, and cranberries. These fruits add interest to muffins, cookies, and other baked goods. If you cannot find the type of dried fruit called for in a recipe, feel free to substitute another type.

Fat-Free Cracker Crumbs. Use fat-free cracker crumbs as a crunchy coating for oven "fried" foods, or as a topping for casseroles. To make this ingredient, simply crush any flavor of fat-free crackers, place in a blender or food processor, and process into crumbs. One ounce of crackers makes about one-fourth cup of crumbs.

Fat-Free Flour and Corn Tortillas. Flour tortillas have always been fairly low in fat, generally with less than 3 grams of fat each. Fat-free brands are now available, as well, and are an even better choice. The recipes in this book use fat-free flour tortillas as wrappers for appetizer finger sandwiches and burritos, and as pizza crusts. If you cannot find a fat-free product, feel free to use regular flour tortillas. Corn tortillas have always been fat-free. Use these handy wrappers to make enchiladas and a variety of other dishes.

Fat-Free Graham Crackers. Graham crackers have always been fairly low in fat, usually with less than 3 grams of fat each. Now that fat-free and low-fat brands are available, though, you have an even healthier option. The recipes in this book use fat-free graham crackers to make graham cracker pie crusts. If you cannot find fat-free grahams, feel free to substitute a regular or low-fat brand.

Fat-Free Granola. A wonderful substitute for nuts, fat-free granola adds nutty crunch and extra flavor to cookies, pancakes, muffins, and other baked goods. Low-fat granola is another good

option. Look for brands with no more than 2 grams of fat per ounce.

Nonstick Cooking Spray. These handy sprays are available both unflavored and in butter and olive oil flavors. While they are pure fat, the amount that comes out of the can during a one-second spray is so small that it adds an insignificant amount of fat to a recipe. In this book, nonstick cooking sprays are used to promote the browning of foods and to prevent foods from sticking to pots and pans.

Olive Oil. While all oils should be limited in a low-fat eating plan, a small amount of olive oil is suggested in an occasional recipe to enhance flavor. When used in the recommended amounts, this ingredient will not blow your fat budget, so include it if you like, using extra virgin olive oil for the most flavor.

What about "light" olive oil? In this case, light refers to flavor—which is mild and bland compared with that of extra virgin oils. This means that you have to use more oil for the same amount of flavor, making this product a poor choice for low-fat cooking.

Sesame Oil. Like olive oil, sesame oil enhances the flavors of foods. Because it is so flavorful, a little bit goes a long way, making this oil a valuable ingredient in low-fat cooking.

Toasted Wheat Germ. This ingredient adds crunch and nutty flavor to baked goods. A super-nutritious food, with 80 percent less fat than nuts, wheat germ provides generous amounts of vitamin E and minerals.

Whole Wheat Bread Crumbs. Whole wheat bread crumbs can be used in stuffings, as a topping for casseroles, or as a filler for meat loaf. To make whole wheat bread crumbs, simply tear up slices of whole wheat bread, place them in a blender or food processor, and process into crumbs. One slice of bread makes about one-half cup of crumbs.

A Word About Salt

Salt, a combination of sodium and chloride, enhances the flavors of many foods. However, most health experts recommend a maximum of 2,400 milligrams of sodium per day, the equivalent of about one teaspoon of salt. For this reason, very little salt is added to the recipes in this book. A minimal use of salt-laden processed ingredients, as well as a wise use of herbs and spices, keeps the salt content under control without compromising taste.

ABOUT THE NUTRITIONAL ANALYSIS

The Food Processor II (ESHA Research) computer nutrition analysis system, along with product information from manufacturers, was used to calculate the nutritional information for the recipes in this book. Nutrients are always listed per one piece, one muffin, one slice of bread, one cookie, one serving, etc.

Sometimes, recipes give you options regarding ingredients. For instance, you might be able to choose between nonfat cream cheese and reduced-fat cream cheese, nonfat mayonnaise and reduced-fat mayonnaise, 96-percent lean ground beef and ground turkey, or raisins and nuts. This will help you create dishes that suit your tastes. Just keep in mind that the nutritional analysis is based on the first ingredient listed.

In your quest for fat-free eating, you might be inclined to choose fat-free cheese over reduced-fat cheese, and to omit any optional nuts. Be aware, though, that if you are not used to nonfat cheeses, it might be wise to start by using reduced-fat products. Should you opt to omit the nuts? Not necessarily. Nuts are high in fat, but they also contain essential minerals and vitamin E. Some studies have even indicated that people who eat nuts as part of a healthy diet have less

heart disease. If you like nuts, feel free to use them in your cooking and baking. In fat-free recipes like the ones in this book, you can afford to add a few nuts or to sometimes choose the higher-fat ingredient.

WHERE DOES THE FAT COME FROM IN FAT-FREE RECIPES?

You may notice that even though a recipe may contain no oil, butter, margarine, nuts, chocolate chips, or other fatty ingredient, it still contains a small amount of fat (less than one gram). This is because many natural ingredients contain some fat. Whole grains, for example, store a small amount of oil in their germ, the center portion of the grain. This oil is very beneficial because it is loaded with vitamin E, an antioxidant. The germ also provides an abundance of vitamins and minerals. Products made from refined grains and refined flours—ingredients that have been stripped of the germ—do have slightly less fat than whole grain versions, but they also have far less nutrients.

Other ingredients, too, naturally contain small amounts of fat. For instance, fruits and vegetables, like grains, contain some oil. And, again, the oil also provides many important nutrients. Olives, nuts, and lean meats also contribute fat to some recipes. However, when used in small quantities, the amount of fat is insignificant. In fact, the majority of recipes in this book contain less than one gram of fat per serving.

This book is filled with recipes that will make any meal of the day special. The dishes are not only easy to make, satisfying, and delicious, but are also foods that you can feel good about serving to your family and friends. So get ready to create some new family favorites, and to experience the pleasures and rewards of cooking without fat.

2. Breakfasts for Champions

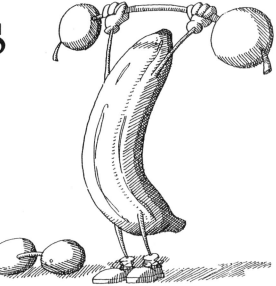

When it comes to high-fat, high-calorie foods, few meals can top a traditional breakfast. For decades, fatty eggs, cheese, sausage, and bacon were considered an essential part of morning fare. Of course, we now know that these foods are far from healthy. But for many of us, breakfast just isn't breakfast without a stack of golden French toast or a hearty Western omelette. What to do, what to do?

Fortunately, you need not discard your favorite breakfast fare in order to banish high-fat foods from the breakfast table. There is now a healthier fat-free or low-fat alternative to just about any breakfast food that comes to mind. Fat-free egg substitutes have been the biggest boon to breakfast lovers. With none of the fat or cholesterol of eggs, these substitutes can replace the eggs in all of your breakfast casseroles and omelettes. Fat-free cheeses and ultra-lean sausage, ham, and bacon are other breakfast favorites that can now take their place in a healthful lifestyle. In fact, many of the recipes in this chapter combine these new fat-free and low-fat ingredients to create delicious versions of previously taboo dishes.

Can pancakes, waffles, and French toast also be part of a low-fat breakfast menu? Happily, many of the traditional recipes for these treats have always been fairly low in fat. However, most recipes do contain unnecessary oil, egg yolks, and salt—unhealthy ingredients that can be trimmed away, leaving these treats just as delicious as always, but a great deal more healthful. Replace the usual refined white flour with whole grain ingredients, add some sweet yet wholesome toppings, and these dishes are more than just low in fat. They are high in many important nutrients.

When creating breakfast menus, you need not confine your choices to the selections in this chapter. Fresh juices, in-season fruits, and whole grain breads and muffins will add both diversity and balance to your menu. So heat up the griddle, and get ready for high-nutrient, taste-tempting breakfast foods that will not only get you out of bed, but will keep you going all morning long!

Banana Granola Pancakes

Yield: 16 pancakes

1½ cups whole wheat flour

1 tablespoon sugar

1 teaspoon baking soda

1¾ cups nonfat buttermilk

2 egg whites, lightly beaten

2 cups sliced bananas (about 2 medium)

½ cup nonfat or low-fat granola cereal

NUTRITIONAL FACTS
(PER PANCAKE)

Calories: 77   Fiber: 1.9 g
Chol: 1 mg   Protein: 3.3 g
Fat: 0.5 g   Sodium: 133 mg

---

1. Combine the flour, sugar, and baking soda in a medium-sized bowl, and stir to mix well. Stir in the buttermilk and egg whites. Fold in the bananas and granola.

2. Coat a griddle or large skillet with nonstick cooking spray, and preheat over medium heat until a drop of water sizzles when it hits the heated surface. (If using an electric griddle, heat the griddle according to the manufacturer's directions.)

3. For each pancake, pour ¼ cup of batter onto the griddle, and spread into a 4-inch circle. Cook for 1 minute and 30 seconds, or until the tops are bubbly and the edges are dry. Turn and cook for an additional minute, or until the second side is golden brown. As the pancakes are done, transfer them to a serving plate and keep warm in a preheated oven.

4. Serve hot, topped with either honey or maple syrup.

Cottage Cheese Pancakes

Yield: 16 pancakes

1 cup whole wheat flour

1 teaspoon dried grated orange rind

1½ teaspoons baking powder

1 cup skim milk

1 cup dry curd or nonfat cottage cheese

4 egg whites, lightly beaten

NUTRITIONAL FACTS
(PER PANCAKE)

Calories: 43   Fiber: 1 g
Chol: 1 mg   Protein: 4 g
Fat: 0.2 g   Sodium: 57 mg

---

1. Combine the whole wheat flour, orange rind, and baking powder in a medium-sized bowl, and stir to mix well. Add the milk, cottage cheese, and egg whites, and stir to mix well.

2. Coat a griddle or large skillet with nonstick cooking spray, and preheat over medium heat until a drop of water sizzles when it hits the heated surface. (If using an electric griddle, heat the griddle according to the manufacturer's directions.)

3. For each pancake, pour 3 tablespoons of batter onto the griddle, and spread into a 3-inch circle. Cook for 1 minute and 30 seconds, or until the tops are bubbly and the edges are dry. Turn and cook for an additional minute, or until the second side is golden brown. As the pancakes are done, transfer them to a serving plate and keep warm in a preheated oven.

4. Serve hot, topped with Berry Fresh Fruit Sauce (page 23) or Honey-Orange Syrup (page 24).

Simple Syrup Alternatives

Deliciously sweet syrups add that crowning touch to pancakes, waffles, and French toast. While all syrups are fat-free, they are generally almost pure sugar, and add up to 60 calories for each tablespoon used. Instead of the usual refined, sugary syrups, try any of the following toppings over pancakes, waffles, and other breakfast treats. As low in calories as most reduced-calorie brands, these syrups are more natural, wholesome, and economical.

Warm Apple Syrup

1. Combine $\frac{3}{4}$ cup of the apple juice and all of the molasses and apples in a 1-quart saucepan. Place over medium heat, and bring to a boil, stirring occasionally. Reduce the heat to low, cover, and simmer for 10 minutes, or until the apples are tender.

2. Combine the cornstarch and the remaining 2 teaspoons of apple juice in a small bowl. Add the mixture to the pan, and cook and stir for 1 minute, or until the mixture is slightly thickened.

3. Serve warm over pancakes, French toast, or waffles. Store any leftovers in the refrigerator for up to a week.

Yield: 1$\frac{3}{4}$ cups

$\frac{3}{4}$ cup plus 2 teaspoons apple juice, divided

$\frac{1}{2}$ cup molasses, honey, or maple syrup

1$\frac{1}{2}$ cups chopped peeled apple (about 2 medium)

2 teaspoons cornstarch

NUTRITIONAL FACTS (PER 2-TABLESPOON SERVING)		
Calories: 50	Fat: 0 g	Protein: 0 g
Cholesterol: 0 mg	Fiber: 0.4 g	Sodium: 5 mg

Berry Fresh Fruit Sauce

1. Combine the sugar and cornstarch in a 1-quart saucepan. Slowly stir in the juice. Place over medium heat, and bring to a boil, stirring constantly.

2. Add the fruit to the juice mixture, and bring to a second boil. Reduce the heat to low, and cook, stirring occasionally, for about 5 minutes, or until the fruit begins to break down and the mixture is thickened and bubbly.

3. Serve warm over pancakes, French toast, or waffles. Store any leftovers in the refrigerator for up to a week.

Yield: 2$\frac{1}{4}$ cups

$\frac{1}{4}$ cup sugar

1 tablespoon cornstarch

$\frac{3}{4}$ cup white grape juice

2 cups fresh or frozen raspberries, blueberries, blackberries, or sliced strawberries

NUTRITIONAL FACTS (PER $\frac{1}{4}$-CUP SERVING)		
Calories: 51	Fat: 0.1 g	Protein: 0.4 g
Cholesterol: 0 mg	Fiber: 1.1 g	Sodium: 1 mg

Honey-Orange Syrup

Yield: 1½ cups

1 tablespoon cornstarch

1 cup orange juice

½ cup honey

1. Combine the cornstarch and orange juice in a 1-quart saucepan, and stir until the cornstarch is dissolved. Stir in the honey.

2. Place the pan over medium heat, and cook and stir for about 3 minutes, or until the mixture is bubbly and slightly thickened.

3. Serve warm over pancakes, French toast, or waffles. Store any leftovers in the refrigerator for up to a week.

NUTRITIONAL FACTS (PER 2-TABLESPOON SERVING)

Calories: 55	Fat: 0 g	Protein: 0.2 g
Cholesterol: 0 mg	Fiber: 0 g	Sodium: 1 mg

Applesauce Pancakes

Yield: 12 pancakes

1½ cups whole wheat flour

1 tablespoon baking powder

¾ cup unsweetened applesauce

1 cup nonfat buttermilk

2 egg whites, lightly beaten

NUTRITIONAL FACTS (PER PANCAKE) ➤

Calories: 69	Fiber: 2 g
Chol: 1 mg	Protein: 3.3 g
Fat: 0.4 g	Sodium: 122 mg

NUTRITIONAL FACTS (PER PANCAKE)

Calories: 69	Fiber: 2 g ➤
Chol: 1 mg	Protein: 3.3 g
Fat: 0.4 g	Sodium: 122 mg

1. Combine the flour and baking powder in a medium-sized bowl, and stir to mix well. Stir in the applesauce, buttermilk, and egg whites.

2. Coat a griddle or large skillet with nonstick cooking spray, and preheat over medium heat until a drop of water sizzles when it hits the heated surface. (If using an electric griddle, heat the griddle according to the manufacturer's directions.)

3. For each pancake, pour ¼ cup of batter onto the griddle, and spread into a 4-inch circle. Cook for 1 minute and 30 seconds, or until the tops are bubbly and the edges are dry. Turn and cook for an additional minute, or until the second side is golden brown. As the pancakes are done, transfer them to a serving plate and keep warm in a preheated oven.

4. Serve hot, topped with Warm Apple Syrup (page 23) or the syrup of your choice.

Variation

To make Applesauce Buckwheat Cakes, substitute ½ cup of buckwheat flour for ½ cup of the whole wheat flour.

Light and Fluffy Oatcakes

Yield: 12 pancakes

1. Combine the oats and buttermilk in a medium-sized bowl. Set aside for 5 minutes.

2. Place the egg whites in the bowl of an electric mixer, and beat on high until stiff peaks form. Set aside.

3. Combine the flour, sugar, and baking powder in a large bowl, and stir to mix well. Add the oat mixture to the flour mixture, and stir to mix well. Gently fold in the egg whites.

4. Coat a griddle or large skillet with nonstick cooking spray, and preheat over medium heat until a drop of water sizzles when it hits the heated surface. (If using an electric griddle, heat the griddle according to the manufacturer's directions.)

5. For each pancake, pour $\frac{1}{4}$ cup of batter onto the griddle, and spread into a 4-inch circle. Cook for 1 minute and 30 seconds, or until the tops are bubbly and the edges are dry. Turn and cook for an additional minute, or until the second side is golden brown. As the pancakes are done, transfer them to a serving plate and keep warm in a preheated oven.

6. Serve hot, topped with Warm Apple Syrup (page 23), Berry Fresh Fruit Sauce (page 23), or Honey-Orange Syrup (page 24).

Variation

To make Blueberry Oatcakes, fold $\frac{3}{4}$ cup of fresh or frozen blueberries into the batter.

¾ cup quick-cooking oats

1¾ cups nonfat buttermilk

2 egg whites

1 cup whole wheat flour

1 tablespoon sugar

2 teaspoons baking powder

NUTRITIONAL FACTS
◄ (PER PANCAKE)

Calories: 75	Fiber: 1.8 g
Chol: 1 mg	Protein: 3.9 g
Fat: 0.8 g	Sodium: 108 mg

NUTRITIONAL FACTS
◄ (PER PANCAKE)

Calories: 80	Fiber: 2 g
Chol: 1 mg	Protein: 4 g
Fat: 0.8 g	Sodium: 108 mg

Golden French Toast

Yield: 12 slices

1. Combine the egg substitute, milk, cinnamon, and vanilla extract in a shallow bowl, and stir to mix well. Dip each slice of bread in the egg mixture, turning to coat both sides.

2. Coat a griddle or large skillet with nonstick cooking spray, and preheat over medium heat until a drop of water sizzles when it hits the heated surface. (If using an electric griddle, heat the griddle according to the manufacturer's directions.)

2 cups fat-free egg substitute

¼ cup skim milk

¼ teaspoon ground cinnamon

1 teaspoon vanilla extract

12 slices whole wheat bread

NUTRITIONAL FACTS
(PER SLICE) ➤

Calories: 82   Fiber: 2 g
Chol: 0 mg   Protein: 8.2 g
Fat: 0.8 g   Sodium: 194 mg

NUTRITIONAL FACTS
(PER SLICE)

Calories: 118   Fiber: 3.3 g
Chol: 0 mg   Protein: 10.9 g ➤
Fat: 1.8 g   Sodium: 194 mg

---

3. Lay the bread slices on the griddle, and cook for about 2 minutes on each side, or until golden brown. As the slices are done, transfer them to a serving plate and keep warm in a preheated oven.

4. Serve hot, either plain or topped with maple syrup, Berry Fresh Fruit Sauce (page 23), or Honey-Orange Syrup (page 24).

Variation

For a crunchy coating, sprinkle each side of the bread with 2 teaspoons of toasted wheat germ just before placing the slice on the griddle.

Crispy Cornmeal Waffles

Yield: 12 waffles

1 cup whole wheat flour
1 cup whole grain cornmeal
2 tablespoons sugar
2 teaspoons baking powder
$\frac{3}{4}$ teaspoon baking soda
4 egg whites
$1\frac{1}{2}$ cups nonfat buttermilk

NUTRITIONAL FACTS
(PER WAFFLE) ➤

Calories: 97   Fiber: 2.0 g
Chol: 0 mg   Protein: 4.3 g
Fat: 0.7 g   Sodium: 194 mg

NUTRITIONAL FACTS
(PER WAFFLE)

Calories: 106   Fiber: 2.3 g
Chol: 0 mg   Protein: 5.1 g ➤
Fat: 1.0 g   Sodium: 194 mg

Waffles are great for people with busy lifestyles, as they may be made in advance, placed in plastic zip-type bags, and frozen until needed. At breakfast time, heat the frozen waffles in the toaster, and serve.

1. Coat a waffle iron with nonstick cooking spray, and preheat according to the manufacturer's directions.

2. Combine the flour, cornmeal, sugar, baking powder, and baking soda in a large bowl, and stir to mix well. Set aside.

3. Place the egg whites in the bowl of an electric mixer, and beat on high until soft peaks form. Set aside.

4. Add the buttermilk to the flour mixture, and stir to mix well. Gently fold in the egg whites.

5. Spoon $1\frac{1}{4}$ cups of batter (or the amount stated by the manufacturer) onto the prepared waffle iron. Bake for 5 to 7 minutes, or until the iron has stopped steaming and the waffle is crisp and brown.

6. Serve hot, topped with Berry Fresh Fruit Sauce (page 23) or Honey-Orange Syrup (page 24).

Variation

For variety and added crunch, fold $\frac{1}{4}$ cup of toasted wheat germ into the batter.

Golden Pumpkin Waffles

1. Coat a waffle iron with nonstick cooking spray, and preheat according to manufacturer's directions.

2. Combine the whole wheat flour, cornmeal or brown rice flour, sugar, baking powder, baking soda, and pumpkin pie spice in a large bowl, and stir to mix well. Set aside.

3. Place the egg whites in the bowl of an electric mixer, and beat on high until soft peaks form. Set aside.

4. Add the pumpkin and milk to the flour mixture, and stir to mix well. Gently fold in the egg whites.

5. Spoon $1\frac{1}{4}$ cups of batter (or the amount stated by the manufacturer) onto the prepared waffle iron. Bake for 6 to 8 minutes, or until the iron has stopped steaming and the waffle is crisp and brown.

6. Serve hot, topped with Warm Apple Syrup (page 23) or Honey-Orange Syrup (page 24).

Yield: 12 waffles

1 cup whole wheat flour

1 cup whole grain cornmeal or brown rice flour

2 tablespoons sugar

2 teaspoons baking powder

$\frac{3}{4}$ teaspoon baking soda

$2\frac{1}{2}$ teaspoons pumpkin pie spice

4 egg whites

$\frac{1}{2}$ cup mashed cooked or canned pumpkin

1 cup skim milk

NUTRITIONAL FACTS
(PER WAFFLE)

Calories: 96	Fiber: 2.2 g
Chol: 0 mg	Protein: 4.1 g
Fat: 0.6 g	Sodium: 172 mg

FAT-FREE COOKING TIP

Getting the Fat Out of Your Waffle Recipes

To make your favorite waffles light, crisp, and fat-free:

- Replace the oil in the recipe with $\frac{3}{4}$ as much buttermilk, applesauce, or other liquid.

- Substitute 3 egg whites for every 2 whole eggs in the recipe, and whip the egg whites to soft peaks before folding them into the batter.

- For an extra-crisp texture, substitute brown rice flour or cornmeal for up to half of the wheat flour. These flours add a pleasing crunch to baked goods.

Spinach and Mushroom Omelette

Yield: 1 serving

¾ cup fat-free egg substitute

⅛ teaspoon ground black pepper

3 tablespoons shredded nonfat
   Cheddar cheese, or 1 slice nonfat
   Cheddar cheese

¼ cup (packed) chopped fresh spinach

2 tablespoons sliced fresh mushrooms

1 slice turkey bacon, cooked, drained,
   and crumbled (optional)

Ground paprika

NUTRITIONAL FACTS
(PER SERVING)

Calories: 125	Fiber: 0.5 g
Chol: 4 mg	Protein: 25 g
Fat: 0.1 g	Sodium: 431 mg

By using fat-free egg substitute instead of whole eggs and nonfat cheese instead of a full-fat product, you will save 235 calories, 25 grams of fat, and 790 milligrams of cholesterol per omelette. Not a bad bargain, considering the great taste of this healthy breakfast dish!

1. Coat an 8-inch nonstick skillet with nonstick cooking spray, and preheat over medium-low heat. Place the egg substitute in the skillet, and sprinkle with the pepper. Let the eggs cook without stirring for about 2 minutes, or until set around the edges.

2. Use a spatula to lift the edges of the omelette, and allow the uncooked egg to flow below the cooked portion. Cook for another minute or 2, or until the eggs are almost set.

3. Arrange first the cheese, and then the spinach, the mushrooms, and, if desired, the bacon over half of the omelette. Fold the other half over the filling, and cook for another minute or 2, or until the cheese is melted and the eggs are completely set.

4. Slide the omelette onto a plate, sprinkle with the paprika, and serve immediately.

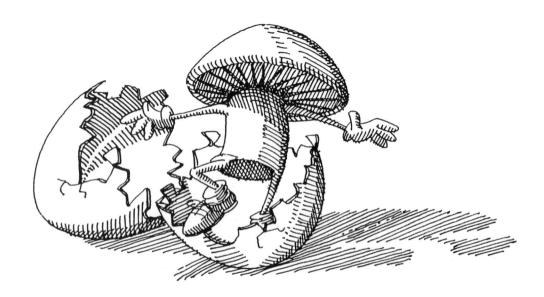

Southwestern Omelette

1. Coat an 8-inch nonstick skillet with nonstick cooking spray, and preheat over medium-low heat. Place the egg substitute in the skillet, and let the eggs cook without stirring for about 2 minutes, or until set around the edges.

2. Use a spatula to lift the edges of the omelette, and allow the uncooked egg to flow below the cooked portion. Cook for another minute or 2, or until the eggs are almost set.

3. Arrange first the cheese, and then the ham, peppers, and onions over half of the omelette. Fold the other half over the filling, and cook for another minute or 2, or until the cheese is melted and the eggs are completely set.

4. Slide the omelette onto a plate, top with the tomatoes or picante sauce, and serve immediately.

Yield: 1 serving

¾ cup fat-free egg substitute

3 tablespoons shredded nonfat Cheddar cheese, or 1 slice nonfat Cheddar cheese

2 tablespoons chopped ham (at least 97% lean)

1 tablespoon chopped green bell pepper

1 tablespoon chopped onion

2 tablespoons chopped tomato or picante sauce

NUTRITIONAL FACTS
(PER SERVING)

Calories: 154	Fiber: 0.5 g
Chol: 14 mg	Protein: 29 g
Fat: 0.7 g	Sodium: 649 mg

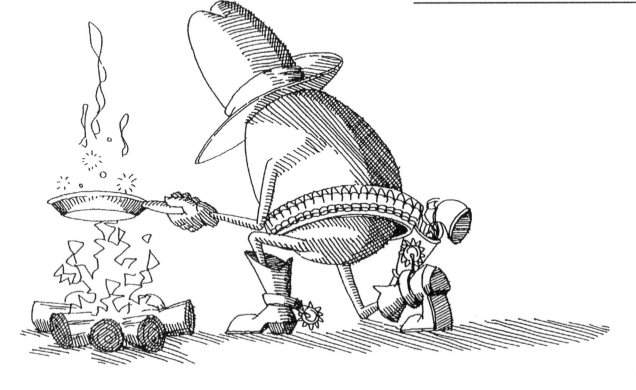

Zucchini Frittata

Yield: 4 servings

1½ medium zucchini, halved lengthwise and sliced ¼ inch thick

1 medium yellow onion, cut into thin wedges

½ medium green bell pepper, cut into thin strips

½ medium red bell pepper, cut into thin strips

1 teaspoon crushed fresh garlic

1 teaspoon dried Italian seasoning

¼ teaspoon ground black pepper

2 cups fat-free egg substitute

¾ cup shredded nonfat or reduced-fat mozzarella cheese

1 tablespoon plus 1½ teaspoons grated nonfat or reduced-fat Parmesan cheese

1. Coat a 10-inch ovenproof skillet with nonstick cooking spray. Place over medium-high heat, and add the zucchini, onions, bell peppers, garlic, Italian seasoning, and black pepper. Cook and stir for 3 minutes, or until the vegetables are crisp-tender.

2. Reduce the heat to low, and pour the egg substitute over the vegetables. Let the eggs cook without stirring for 10 to 12 minutes, or until almost set.

3. Remove the skillet from the heat, and place under a preheated broiler. Broil 6 inches from the heat for about 3 minutes, or until the eggs are set.

4. Sprinkle the cheeses over the frittata, and broil for an additional minute, or just until the cheese has melted. Cut the frittata into wedges, and serve immediately.

NUTRITIONAL FACTS (PER SERVING)		
Calories: 119	Fat: 0.1 g	Protein: 20.6 g
Cholesterol: 6 mg	Fiber: 1.5 g	Sodium: 370 mg

Fruit Muesli

Yield: 5 cups

2 cups old-fashioned oats

¼ cup plus 2 tablespoons wheat bran

¾ cup barley nugget cereal

¼ cup toasted wheat germ

½ cup dark raisins or chopped dates

½ cup chopped dried apricots

½ cup chopped dried peaches

½ cup chopped pecans, hazelnuts, walnuts, or almonds (optional)

This supernutritious breakfast cereal is a snap to make.

1. Place all of the ingredients in a large bowl, and stir to mix well. Transfer to an airtight container, and store for up to 4 weeks.

2. To serve, place ⅓ cup of museli in an individual serving bowl, and add ½ cup of low-fat milk, nonfat vanilla or plain yogurt, or applesauce. Stir, and let sit for 3 to 5 minutes before serving.

NUTRITIONAL FACTS (PER ⅓-CUP SERVING, CEREAL ONLY)		
Calories: 108	Fat: 1 g	Protein: 3.7 g
Cholesterol: 0 mg	Fiber: 3.4 g	Sodium: 40 mg

Potato-Crusted Sausage Quiche

1. Combine the egg substitute, cottage cheese, flour, pepper, and Tabasco sauce in a large bowl, and stir to mix well. Stir in the cheese, sausage, and scallions. Set aside.

2. Coat a 9-inch deep dish pie pan with nonstick cooking spray. Slice the unpeeled potatoes $\frac{1}{4}$ inch thick, and arrange the slices in a single layer over the bottom and sides of the pan to form a crust. Pour the egg mixture into the crust.

3. Bake uncovered at 375°F for 45 minutes, or until a sharp knife inserted in the center of the quiche comes out clean. Allow to cool at room temperature for 5 minutes before cutting into wedges and serving.

Yield: 5 servings

1 cup fat-free egg substitute

1 cup dry curd or low-fat cottage cheese

1 tablespoon unbleached flour

$\frac{1}{8}$ teaspoon ground black pepper

$\frac{1}{2}$ teaspoon Tabasco pepper sauce

1 cup shredded nonfat or reduced-fat Cheddar cheese

4 ounces smoked turkey sausage (at least 97% lean), diced

2 scallions, finely chopped

2 medium potatoes, scrubbed

NUTRITIONAL FACTS (PER SERVING)

Calories: 190	Fat: 0.6 g	Protein: 22 g
Cholesterol: 16 mg	Fiber: 1.8 g	Sodium: 489 mg

Ham and Cheese Breakfast Biscuits

1. Combine the flour, oat bran, and baking powder in a medium-sized bowl, and stir to mix well. Add the buttermilk, and stir to mix well. Fold in the cheese and ham.

2. Coat a 9-inch round pan with nonstick cooking spray. Drop heaping tablespoonfuls of the batter onto the pan, spacing the biscuits 1 inch apart.

3. Bake at 400°F for 20 minutes, or until lightly browned. Transfer to a serving platter, and serve hot.

Yield: 8 biscuits

1 cup unbleached flour

$\frac{1}{2}$ cup oat bran

2 teaspoons baking powder

$\frac{3}{4}$ cup nonfat buttermilk

$\frac{1}{2}$ cup shredded nonfat or reduced-fat Cheddar cheese

2 ounces ham (at least 97% lean), finely chopped

NUTRITIONAL FACTS (PER BISCUIT)

Calories: 98	Fat: 0.9 g	Protein: 6.7 g
Cholesterol: 5 mg	Fiber: 1.4 g	Sodium: 231 mg

Eggchiladas

Yield: 4 servings

8 corn tortillas (6-inch rounds)

1 cup shredded nonfat or reduced-fat Cheddar cheese

FILLING

1 cup diced cooked potato

$\frac{1}{4}$ cup chopped green bell pepper

$\frac{1}{4}$ cup chopped onion

$\frac{1}{2}$ teaspoon whole cumin seed

$\frac{1}{4}$ teaspoon ground black pepper

2 cups fat-free egg substitute

SAUCE

1 can (8 ounces) unsalted tomato sauce

1 cup water, divided

1 tablespoon chili powder

1 tablespoon plus $1\frac{1}{2}$ teaspoons unbleached flour

NUTRITIONAL FACTS
(PER SERVING)

Calories: 265	Fiber: 4.2 g
Chol: 5 mg	Protein: 25 g
Fat: 0.8 g	Sodium: 235 mg

1. To make the filling, coat a large nonstick skillet with nonstick cooking spray, and preheat over medium-high heat. Add the potatoes, bell peppers, onions, cumin, and black pepper, and cook and stir for 2 to 3 minutes, or until the peppers and onions are crisp-tender.

2. Reduce the heat to medium-low, and add the egg substitute. Cook for 2 minutes without stirring. Then, stirring gently to scramble, cook for 2 additional minutes, or just until the eggs are cooked through. Remove the skillet from the heat, cover to keep warm, and set aside.

3. To make the sauce, place the tomato sauce, $\frac{3}{4}$ cup of the water, and the chili powder in an 8-inch skillet. (Note that this must be cooked in a skillet, rather than a saucepan, because you will later dip the tortillas in the sauce.) Place over medium heat, and bring to a boil.

4. Combine the flour and the remaining $\frac{1}{4}$ cup of water in a jar with a tight-fitting lid, and shake until smooth. Slowly add the flour mixture to the tomato sauce, stirring constantly, and cook until bubbly. Reduce the heat to low to keep the sauce warm.

5. Coat a 9-x-13-inch baking dish with nonstick cooking spray, and set aside. Using tongs, dip a tortilla in the warm sauce for 5 to 10 seconds, coating both sides, to soften. Lay the tortilla on a flat surface, and spoon $\frac{1}{3}$ cup of the filling along the bottom. Roll the tortilla up to enclose the filling, and place seam side down in the prepared dish. Repeat with the remaining tortillas, leaving about $\frac{1}{8}$ inch of space between the tortillas for easy serving.

6. Pour the remaining sauce over the filled tortillas, and sprinkle with the cheese. Bake at 375°F for 10 to 12 minutes, or until the dish is heated through and the cheese is melted. Serve immediately.

Hot Apple Kasha

1. Combine the millet and water in a 1½-quart saucepan, and bring to a boil over high heat. Reduce the heat to low, cover, and simmer for 15 minutes without stirring.

2. Combine the buckwheat and cinnamon in a small bowl, and add the mixture to the pot. Stir in the apple juice and chopped apple. Cover and cook, without stirring, for 10 minutes, or until the liquid has been absorbed and the grains are tender.

3. Remove the pot from the heat and let sit, covered, for 5 minutes. Serve hot, plain or with a topping of maple syrup and skim milk.

Yield: 4 servings

½ cup uncooked millet

1¼ cups water

¼ cup uncooked roasted buckwheat kernels (kasha)

¼ teaspoon ground cinnamon

1 cup apple juice

1 medium apple, peeled and coarsely chopped

NUTRITIONAL FACTS (PER ¾-CUP SERVING)		
Calories: 156	Fat: 0.9 g	Protein: 3.2 g
Cholesterol: 0 mg	Fiber: 3 g	Sodium: 4 mg

Bulgur Wheat Breakfast

1. Combine all of the ingredients in a 1½-quart saucepan, and bring to a boil over high heat. Reduce the heat to low, cover, and simmer for 5 minutes without stirring.

2. Remove the pot from the heat and let sit, covered, for 15 to 20 minutes, or until the liquid has been absorbed and the grains are tender. Serve hot, plain or topped with honey and skim milk.

Yield: 5 servings

1 cup uncooked bulgur wheat

3 tablespoons toasted wheat germ

⅓ cup chopped dried apricots

⅓ cup chopped prunes

2½ cups water

NUTRITIONAL FACTS (PER ¾-CUP SERVING)		
Calories: 160	Fat: 0.9 g	Protein: 5.3 g
Cholesterol: 0 mg	Fiber: 7.4 g	Sodium: 6 mg

3. Bountiful Breads

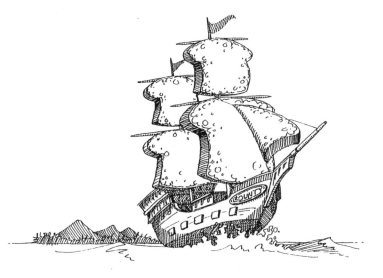

Nothing warms the heart and tempts the taste buds like the smell of fresh-baked breads, rolls, muffins, and biscuits. Until very recently, though, most muffins, quick breads, and other baked goods were made with large amounts of butter, margarine, oil, and other high-fat ingredients—ingredients that must be kept to a minimum in a healthy diet. Fortunately, times have changed, and we now know that delicious baked goods can be made with little or no fat.

Most breads are simple to make, and when you bake your own, you can not only reduce or eliminate the fat, but also boost the nutritional value of your product by using a variety of whole grain flours and by reducing the amount of sugar used. In fact, the baked goods recipes in this book contain 25 to 50 percent less sugar than traditional recipes do. Naturally sweet and flavorful ingredients like fruit juices, fruit purées, and oats reduce the need for sugar while enhancing the taste and aroma of your home-baked treats.

Will your baked goods be dry if you leave out the oil and butter? Not if you replace the fat with fruit juices, fruit purées, nonfat buttermilk, and other healthful fat substitutes. The recipes in this chapter combine these natural substitutes with whole grain flours to produce an array of super-moist, tempting breads. From Jalapeño Cornbread to Apple Butter Bread to Very Blueberry Muffins, you'll find breads for every meal of the day. Just as important, you'll learn how to apply the secrets of fat-free baking to your own recipes so that you and your family can enjoy new, healthful versions of old family favorites.

Before mixing up the batter for your first fat-free muffin or loaf, you may want to turn to "About the Ingredients," on page 5. That section will acquaint you with the whole grain flours you'll be using, and will guide you in substituting less-refined sweeteners for traditional sweeteners, if you wish to do so. Then take out your baking pans, preheat your oven, and get ready to create some of the healthiest, most flavorful breads you've ever tasted!

Broccoli Cheese Muffins

Yield: 16 muffins

2 cups whole grain cornmeal

1 tablespoon sugar

1 tablespoon baking powder

½ teaspoon baking soda

1½ cups nonfat buttermilk

3 egg whites, lightly beaten

1 package (10 ounces) frozen chopped broccoli, thawed and squeezed dry

1 cup shredded nonfat or reduced-fat Cheddar cheese

1. Combine the cornmeal, sugar, baking powder, and baking soda in a large bowl, and stir to mix well. Add the buttermilk and egg whites, and stir just until the dry ingredients are moistened. Fold in the broccoli and cheese.

2. Coat muffin cups with cooking spray, and fill ¾ full with the batter. Bake at 350°F for 16 to 18 minutes, or just until a wooden toothpick inserted in the center of a muffin comes out clean.

3. Remove the muffin tins from the oven, and allow them to sit for 5 minutes before removing the muffins. Serve warm.

NUTRITIONAL FACTS (PER MUFFIN)

Calories: 86	Fat: 0.8 g	Protein: 5.4 g
Cholesterol: 2 mg	Fiber: 1.7 g	Sodium: 202 mg

Cranberry Apple Muffins

Yield: 12 muffins

2 cups whole wheat flour

¼ cup plus 2 tablespoons sugar

1 tablespoon baking powder

¼ teaspoon baking soda

½ teaspoon ground cinnamon

¾ cup plus 2 tablespoons apple juice

2 egg whites, lightly beaten

1 cup finely chopped apple (about 1½ medium)

⅓ cup coarsely chopped fresh or frozen cranberries

⅓ cup golden raisins

1. Combine the flour, sugar, baking powder, baking soda, and cinnamon in a large bowl, and stir to mix well. Add the apple juice, egg whites, and chopped apples, and stir just until the dry ingredients are moistened. Fold in the cranberries and raisins.

2. Coat muffin cups with cooking spray, and fill ¾ full with the batter. Bake at 350°F for 16 minutes, or just until a wooden toothpick inserted in the center of a muffin comes out clean.

3. Remove the muffin tins from the oven, and allow them to sit for 5 minutes before removing the muffins. Serve warm or at room temperature.

NUTRITIONAL FACTS (PER MUFFIN)

Calories: 124	Fat: 0.4 g	Protein: 3.5 g
Cholesterol: 0 mg	Fiber: 2.9 g	Sodium: 128 mg

Getting the Fat Out of Your Muffin, Quick Bread, and Cake Recipes

As the recipes in this chapter illustrate, almost any moist ingredient can replace the fat in muffins, breads, and biscuits, as well as other baked goods. It is important to realize, though, that some recipes are better candidates for fat reduction than others. Quick breads and muffins are some of the most easily adapted recipes. Coffee cakes, carrot cakes, spice cakes, and those yeast breads that naturally have denser textures are also easily made fat-free. Any cakes and other baked goods that are meant to have a very light, tender texture are the most difficult to modify. However, you can easily eliminate one-half to three-fourths of the fat even in these recipes.

When you modify your recipes, try eliminating only half the fat at first. The next time you make the recipe, try replacing even more of the fat. Whenever you *completely* eliminate the fat from a recipe, it is best to substitute whole wheat flour for at least one-third of the white flour, or to substitute oat bran for one-fourth of the white flour. This will help maintain a pleasing texture.

As you begin working with fat substitutes, you will learn that each type of fat substitute has its own set of "rules"—guidelines that will allow you to successfully modify your particular recipe. For instance, it is usually necessary to lower the oven temperature, as fat-free products can become dry if baked in an overly hot oven. The remainder of this inset will look at the many available fat substitutes, and will guide you in using these substitutes to "defat" favorite muffin, quick bread, and cake recipes. For guidelines on modifying cookie and brownie recipes, see the inset on page 170.

Using Fat Substitutes in Muffins, Quick Breads, and Cakes

Fat Substitutes	In Which Items Do These Work Best?	How Should Your Recipes Be Modified When Using These Fat Substitutes?
Applesauce, mashed banana, puréed fruits, fruit juice, nonfat buttermilk, nonfat yogurt, and skim milk.	Use applesauce, nonfat buttermilk, nonfat yogurt, or skim milk to make biscuits, muffins, chocolate cakes, and other baked goods whose flavor you do not want to change. Use fruit juices and purées in carrot and spice cakes, breads, and muffins.	• Replace part or all of the butter, margarine, or other solid fat in muffins, breads, biscuits, scones, and cakes with half as much fat substitute. Replace part or all of the oil with three-fourths as much fat substitute. Mix up the batter, and add more substitute if the batter seems too dry. • Replace each whole egg with one egg white. • Reduce the oven temperature by 25°F. • Check for doneness a few minutes before the end of the usual baking time.

Fat Substitutes	In Which Items Do These Work Best?	How Should Your Recipes Be Modified When Using These Fat Substitutes?
Honey, maple syrup, corn syrup, chocolate syrup, fruit jams and spreads, and fruit juice concentrates.	Use honey or fruit jam in muffins; maple syrup in spice cakes and muffins; fruit juice concentrates in muffins and breads; corn syrup in white cakes and other baked goods whose flavor you do not want to change; and chocolate syrup in chocolate cakes and other chocolate treats.	• Replace part or all of the butter, margarine, or other solid fat in muffins, breads, scones, and cakes with three-fourths as much fat substitute. Replace part or all of the oil with an equal amount of fat substitute. Mix up the batter, and add more substitute if the batter seems too dry. • Replace each whole egg with one egg white. • Reduce the sugar by the amount of fat substitute being added. • Reduce the oven temperature by 25°F. • Check for doneness a few minutes before the end of the usual baking time.
Prune Butter (page 160)	This substitute is delicious in chocolate cakes and in fruit- or spice-flavored muffins, breads, and cakes.	• Replace part or all of the butter, margarine, or other solid fat in muffins, breads, scones, and cakes with an equal amount of Prune Butter. • Replace each whole egg with one egg white. • Reduce the sugar by one-half to two-thirds the amount of Prune Butter being added. • Reduce the oven temperature by 25°F. • Check for doneness a few minutes before the end of the usual baking time.
Prune Purée (page 160)	Because of Prune Purée's mild flavor, it works well in all recipes.	• Replace part or all of the butter, margarine, or other solid fat in muffins, breads, scones, and cakes with half as much Prune Purée. Replace part or all of the oil with three-fourths as much of the purée. Mix up the batter, and add more substitute if the batter seems too dry. • Replace each whole egg with one egg white *or* two additional tablespoons of Prune Purée. • Reduce the oven temperature by 25°F. • Check for doneness a few minutes before the end of the usual baking time.

Fat Substitutes	In Which Items Do These Work Best?	How Should Your Recipes Be Modified When Using These Fat Substitutes?
Mashed cooked or canned pumpkin, butternut squash, and sweet potatoes.	Use these substitutes in biscuits, muffins, breads, and spice cakes. They work particularly well in citrus- and pineapple-flavored baked goods.	• Replace part or all of the butter, margarine, or other solid fat in muffins, breads, scones, biscuits, and cakes with three-fourths as much fat substitute. Replace part or all of the oil with an equal amount of fat substitute. Mix up the batter, and add more substitute if the batter seems too dry. • Replace each whole egg with one egg white. • Reduce the oven temperature by 25°F. • Check for doneness a few minutes before the end of the usual baking time.

Banana Oat Bran Muffins

1. Combine the topping ingredients in a small bowl. Stir to mix well, and set aside.

2. Combine the flour, oat bran, sugar, baking powder, baking soda, and nutmeg in a large bowl, and stir to mix well. Add the mashed bananas, juice, and egg whites, and stir just until the dry ingredients are moistened. Fold in the dates or apricots.

3. Coat muffin cups with cooking spray, and fill $^3/_4$ full with the batter. Sprinkle $^1/_2$ teaspoon of the topping over each muffin, and bake at 350°F for 16 to 18 minutes, or just until a wooden toothpick inserted in the center of a muffin comes out clean.

4. Remove the muffin tins from the oven, and allow them to sit for 5 minutes before removing the muffins. Serve warm or at room temperature.

Yield: 12 muffins

1½ cups whole wheat flour

¾ cup oat bran

¼ cup light brown sugar

1 tablespoon baking powder

¼ teaspoon baking soda

¼ teaspoon ground nutmeg

1½ cups mashed very ripe banana (about 3 large)

¼ cup pineapple or orange juice

2 egg whites, lightly beaten

⅓ cup chopped dates or dried apricots

TOPPING

1 tablespoon finely chopped walnuts

1 tablespoon light brown sugar

NUTRITIONAL FACTS (PER MUFFIN)

Calories: 131	Fat: 1 g	Protein: 4.1 g
Cholesterol: 0 mg	Fiber: 3.7 g	Sodium: 128 mg

Honey Bran Muffins

Yield: 12 muffins

1 cup wheat bran

1¼ cups plus 2 tablespoons nonfat buttermilk

1½ cups whole wheat flour

1 teaspoon baking soda

¼ cup plus 2 tablespoons honey

2 egg whites, lightly beaten

½ cup chopped dried apricots or prunes

1. Combine the bran and buttermilk in a medium-sized bowl. Stir to mix well, and set aside for 15 minutes.

2. Combine the flour and baking soda in a large bowl, and stir to mix well. Add the bran mixture, honey, and egg whites, and stir just until the dry ingredients are moistened. Fold in the apricots or prunes.

3. Coat muffin cups with cooking spray, and fill ¾ full with the batter. Bake at 350°F for 16 minutes, or just until a wooden toothpick inserted in the center of a muffin comes out clean.

4. Remove the muffin tins from the oven, and allow them to sit for 5 minutes before removing the muffins. Serve warm or at room temperature.

NUTRITIONAL FACTS (PER MUFFIN)

Calories: 120	Fat: 0.7 g	Protein: 4.5 g
Cholesterol: 0 mg	Fiber: 4.3 g	Sodium: 145 mg

Fresh Pear Muffins

Yield: 12 muffins

1½ cups whole wheat flour

¾ cup oat bran

⅓ cup sugar

1 tablespoon baking powder

¼ teaspoon ground cinnamon

¼ teaspoon ground nutmeg

1 cup pear nectar

2 egg whites, lightly beaten

¾ cup finely chopped pear (about 1 medium)

¼ cup dark raisins or chopped walnuts

1. Combine the flour, oat bran, sugar, baking powder, cinnamon, and nutmeg in a large bowl, and stir to mix well. Add the nectar, egg whites, and chopped pear, and stir just until the dry ingredients are moistened. Fold in the raisins or walnuts.

2. Coat muffin cups with cooking spray, and fill ¾ full with the batter. Bake at 350°F for 15 to 17 minutes, or just until a wooden toothpick inserted in the center of a muffin comes out clean.

3. Remove the muffin tins from the oven, and allow them to sit for 5 minutes before removing the muffins. Serve warm or at room temperature.

NUTRITIONAL FACTS (PER MUFFIN)

Calories: 121	Fat: 0.7 g	Protein: 3.8 g
Cholesterol: 0 mg	Fiber: 3.3 g	Sodium: 102 mg

Top Left: Ham and Cheese Breakfast Biscuits (page 31)
Top Right: Golden French Toast (page 25)
Bottom: Crispy Cornmeal Waffles (page 26)

Top Left: Carrot Raisin Bread (page 44)
Top Right: Broccoli Cheese Muffins (page 36)
Bottom: Applesauce Sticky Buns (page 48)

Top: Fiesta Roll-Ups (page 57)
Center: Stuffed Finger Sandwiches (page 56)
Bottom: Shrimp Bruschetta (page 52)

Top Left: Zippy Artichoke Dip (page 59)
Top Right: Aloha Meatballs (page 54)
Bottom Left: Crab-Stuffed Mushrooms (page 53)
Bottom Right: Chicken Fingers With Sauce (page 55)

Very Blueberry Muffins

For variety, substitute coarsely chopped raspberries, black-berries, or sweet pitted cherries for the blueberries.

1. Combine the oats, yogurt, and orange juice in a medium-sized bowl. Stir to mix well, and set aside for 5 minutes.

2. Combine the flour, sugar, baking powder, baking soda, and orange rind in a large bowl, and stir to mix well. Add the oat mixture and egg whites, and stir just until the dry ingredients are moistened. Fold in the blueberries.

3. Coat muffin cups with cooking spray, and fill ¾ full with the batter. Sprinkle ¼ teaspoon of sugar over the top of each muffin, and bake at 350°F for 16 minutes, or just until a wooden toothpick inserted in the center of a muffin comes out clean.

4. Remove the muffin tins from the oven, and allow them to sit for 5 minutes before removing the muffins. Serve warm or at room temperature.

Yield: 12 muffins

1¼ cups quick-cooking oats

¾ cup plain nonfat yogurt

½ cup orange juice

1¼ cups whole wheat flour

⅓ cup sugar

1 tablespoon baking powder

¼ teaspoon baking soda

1 teaspoon dried grated orange rind, or 1 tablespoon fresh

2 egg whites, lightly beaten

1 cup fresh or frozen blueberries

TOPPING

1 tablespoon sugar

NUTRITIONAL FACTS (PER MUFFIN)

Calories: 123	Fat: 0.8 g	Protein: 4.7 g
Cholesterol: 0 mg	Fiber: 2.8 g	Sodium: 140 mg

Tips for Super-Moist Fat-Free Baking

The most common complaint people have about fat-free baked goods is that they are too dry. The good news is that it is possible to produce deliciously moist fat-free muffins, quick breads, cakes, and other baked goods. Here are some important tips that you should keep in mind whenever you bake fat-free treats.

❑ *Avoid overbaking.* Fat-free treats bake more quickly than do those made with fat. Baked at too high a temperature or left in the oven too long, they will become dry. That's why the recipes in this book recommend lower-than-standard oven temperatures and shorter-than-standard baking times.

❑ *Use the toothpick test or another test of doneness.* The best way to check fat-free muffins, quick breads, and cakes for doneness is to do the toothpick test. Insert a wooden toothpick in the center of the product. When the toothpick comes out clean, the product should be removed from the oven. When using one of this book's cookie or brownie recipes, use the test of doneness provided in that recipe.

❑ *Keep your baked goods moist and fresh.* Fat-free baked goods made with the natural fat substitutes suggested in this book will have a high moisture content and no preservatives. It is a good idea to refrigerate any quick breads, muffins, and cakes not eaten within twenty-four hours. The recipes will let you know when a product must be refrigerated immediately after baking.

Oatmeal, Fruit, and Nut Bread

Yield: 16 slices

¾ cup quick-cooking oats

1¼ cups nonfat buttermilk

1½ cups whole wheat flour

½ cup light brown sugar

1 teaspoon baking powder

1 teaspoon baking soda

2 teaspoons vanilla extract

⅓ cup dried cherries, blueberries, cranberries, or raisins

¼ cup chopped pecans

1. Combine the oats and buttermilk in a medium-sized bowl. Stir to mix well, and set aside.

2. Combine the flour, brown sugar, baking powder, and baking soda in a large bowl, and stir to mix well, pressing out any lumps. Add the buttermilk mixture and vanilla, and stir just until the dry ingredients are moistened. Fold in the fruits and nuts.

3. Coat an 8-x-4-inch loaf pan with cooking spray. Spread the batter in the pan, and bake at 325°F for 35 minutes, or just until a toothpick inserted in the center of the loaf comes out clean.

4. Remove the bread from the oven, and let sit for 10 minutes. Turn the loaf onto a wire rack, and cool before slicing.

NUTRITIONAL FACTS (PER SLICE)		
Calories: 100	Fat: 1.9 g	Protein: 3 g
Cholesterol: 0 mg	Fiber: 2 g	Sodium: 124 mg

Pumpkin Perfection Bread

Yield: 16 slices

1⅔ cups whole wheat flour

½ cup sugar

1 teaspoon baking powder

1 teaspoon baking soda

2 teaspoons pumpkin pie spice

1 cup mashed cooked or canned pumpkin

¼ cup plus 2 tablespoons orange juice

¼ cup Prune Purée (page 160)

¼ cup toasted wheat germ or chopped pecans

1. Combine the flour, sugar, baking powder, baking soda, and pumpkin pie spice in a large bowl, and stir to mix well. Add the pumpkin, orange juice, and Prune Purée, and stir just until the dry ingredients are moistened. Fold in the wheat germ or pecans.

2. Coat an 8-x-4-inch loaf pan with nonstick cooking spray. Spread the batter evenly in the pan, and bake at 325°F for 40 to 45 minutes, or just until a wooden toothpick inserted in the center of the loaf comes out clean.

3. Remove the bread from the oven, and let sit for 10 minutes. Turn the loaf onto a wire rack, and cool before slicing.

NUTRITIONAL FACTS (PER SLICE)		
Calories: 84	Fat: 0.5 g	Protein: 2.5 g
Cholesterol: 0 mg	Fiber: 2.3 g	Sodium: 103 mg

Raisin Bran Bread

Yield: 16 slices

1⅔ cups whole wheat flour

1¼ cups wheat bran

1 teaspoon baking soda

1⅓ cups skim milk

⅓ cup molasses

1 tablespoon lemon juice

⅓ cup dark raisins

1. Combine the flour, wheat bran, and baking soda in a large bowl, and stir to mix well. Set aside.

2. Combine the milk, molasses, and lemon juice in a medium-sized bowl, and stir to mix well. Add the milk mixture to the flour mixture, and stir just until the dry ingredients are moistened. Fold in the raisins.

3. Coat an 8-x-4-inch loaf pan with nonstick cooking spray. Spread the batter evenly in the pan, and bake at 350°F for 35 minutes, or just until a wooden toothpick inserted in the center of the loaf comes out clean.

4. Remove the bread from the oven, and let sit for 10 minutes. Turn the loaf onto a wire rack, and cool before slicing.

NUTRITIONAL FACTS (PER SLICE)

Calories: 88	Fat: 0.5 g	Protein: 3.2 g
Cholesterol: 0 mg	Fiber: 3.6 g	Sodium: 93 mg

Apple Butter Bread

Yield: 16 slices

2 cups whole wheat flour

1 teaspoon baking powder

1 teaspoon baking soda

¼ teaspoon ground nutmeg

1 cup apple butter

½ cup plus 2 tablespoons apple juice

1 teaspoon vanilla extract

½ cup dark raisins or currants

¼ cup chopped walnuts (optional)

1. Combine the flour, baking powder, baking soda, and nutmeg in a large bowl, and stir to mix well. Add the apple butter, apple juice, and vanilla extract, and stir just until the dry ingredients are moistened. Fold in the raisins or currants and, if desired, the walnuts.

2. Coat an 8-x-4-inch loaf pan with nonstick cooking spray. Spread the batter evenly in the pan, and bake at 350°F for 40 to 45 minutes, or just until a wooden toothpick inserted in the center of the loaf comes out clean.

3. Remove the bread from the oven, and let sit for 10 minutes. Turn the loaf onto a wire rack, and cool before slicing.

NUTRITIONAL FACTS (PER SLICE)

Calories: 103	Fat: 0.3 g	Protein: 2.2 g
Cholesterol: 0 mg	Fiber: 2.2 g	Sodium: 103 mg

Pineapple-Poppy Seed Bread

Yield: 16 slices

2 cups whole wheat flour

⅓ cup sugar

1 teaspoon baking powder

1 teaspoon baking soda

1 can (8 ounces) crushed pineapple in juice, undrained

⅓ cup skim milk

1 teaspoon vanilla extract

½ teaspoon almond extract

2 tablespoons poppy seeds

1. Combine the flour, sugar, baking powder, and baking soda in a large bowl, and stir to mix well. Add the pineapple, including the juice, and the milk and extracts, and stir just until the dry ingredients are moistened. Fold in the poppy seeds.

2. Coat an 8-x-4-inch loaf pan with nonstick cooking spray. Spread the batter evenly in the pan, and bake at 350°F for 40 minutes, or just until a wooden toothpick inserted in the center of the loaf comes out clean.

3. Remove the bread from the oven, and let sit for 10 minutes. Turn the loaf onto a wire rack, and cool before slicing.

NUTRITIONAL FACTS (PER SLICE)

Calories: 83	Fat: 0.8 g	Protein: 2.5 g
Cholesterol: 0 mg	Fiber: 2.1 g	Sodium: 105 mg

Carrot Raisin Bread

Yield: 16 slices

2 cups whole wheat flour

½ cup sugar

1 teaspoon baking powder

1 teaspoon baking soda

1 teaspoon ground cinnamon

1 cup apple or orange juice

1 cup finely grated carrots (about 2 medium)

⅓ cup dark or golden raisins

¼ cup toasted wheat germ

1. Combine the flour, sugar, baking powder, baking soda, and cinnamon in a large bowl, and stir to mix well. Add the juice and carrots, and stir just until the dry ingredients are moistened. Fold in the raisins and wheat germ.

2. Coat an 8-x-4-inch loaf pan with nonstick cooking spray. Spread the batter evenly in the pan, and bake at 350°F for 45 minutes, or just until a wooden toothpick inserted in the center of the loaf comes out clean.

3. Remove the bread from the oven, and let sit for 10 minutes. Turn the loaf onto a wire rack, and cool before slicing.

NUTRITIONAL FACTS (PER SLICE)

Calories: 102	Fat: 0.5 g	Protein: 2.8 g
Cholesterol: 0 mg	Fiber: 2.4 g	Sodium: 105 mg

Jalapeño Cornbread

1. Combine the cornmeal, flour, sugar, baking powder, and baking soda in a large bowl, and stir to mix well. Add the buttermilk and egg whites, and stir just until the dry ingredients are moistened. Fold in the corn, cheese, and jalapeños.

2. Coat a 10-inch ovenproof skillet with nonstick cooking spray, and spread the batter evenly in the pan. Bake at 350°F for 25 to 30 minutes, or just until a wooden toothpick inserted in the center of the bread comes out clean.

3. Remove the bread from the oven, and let it sit for 5 minutes. Cut the bread into wedges, and serve hot.

Yield: 12 servings

1¼ cups whole grain cornmeal

¾ cup whole wheat flour

1 tablespoon sugar

2 teaspoons baking powder

½ teaspoon baking soda

1½ cups nonfat buttermilk

2 egg whites, lightly beaten

¾ cup fresh or frozen (thawed) whole kernel corn

½ cup shredded nonfat or reduced-fat Cheddar cheese

1–2 tablespoons finely chopped jalapeño peppers

NUTRITIONAL FACTS (PER SERVING)

Calories: 106	Fat: 0.8 g	Protein: 5.5 g
Cholesterol: 2 mg	Fiber: 2.1 g	Sodium: 202 mg

Buttermilk Drop Biscuits

1. Combine the flour, oat bran, sugar, and baking powder in a large bowl, and stir to mix well. Add the buttermilk, and stir just until the dry ingredients are moistened. Add a little more buttermilk if needed to form a stiff batter.

2. Coat a baking sheet with nonstick cooking spray, and drop heaping tablespoonfuls of the batter onto the sheet. For crusty biscuits, space the spoonfuls 1 inch apart; for soft biscuits, space the spoonfuls so that they are barely touching.

3. Bake at 400°F for 18 minutes, or just until the tops are lightly browned. Transfer to a serving plate, and serve hot.

Yield: 12 biscuits

2 cups unbleached flour

½ cup oat bran

1 tablespoon sugar

1 tablespoon baking powder

1¼ cups plus 2 tablespoons nonfat buttermilk

NUTRITIONAL FACTS (PER BISCUIT)

Calories: 101	Fat: 0.7 g	Protein: 3.7 g
Cholesterol: 0 mg	Fiber: 1.3 g	Sodium: 121 mg

Prune-Filled Tea Bread

Yield: 16 slices

DOUGH

2 cups unbleached flour

3 tablespoons sugar

2 teaspoons Rapid Rise yeast

½ teaspoon salt

¾ cup skim milk

1 egg white

¾ cup whole wheat flour

2 teaspoons skim milk or beaten egg white

FILLING

1 cup chopped prunes

1 cup white grape juice

GLAZE

⅓ cup confectioner's sugar

1¼ teaspoons white grape juice

¼ teaspoon almond extract

NUTRITIONAL FACTS (PER SLICE)

Calories: 135	Fiber: 2.2 g
Chol: 0 mg	Protein: 3.4 g
Fat: 0.3 g	Sodium: 78 mg

For variety, substitute chopped dried apricots for the prunes.

1. To prepare the filling, combine the prunes and juice in a 1-quart saucepan, and bring to a boil over high heat. Reduce the heat to low, cover, and simmer for 15 to 20 minutes, or until the prunes have absorbed the liquid. Remove the pot from the heat, and let the mixture cool to room temperature.

2. To make the dough, combine the unbleached flour with the sugar, yeast, and salt in a large bowl. Stir to mix well, and set aside.

3. Place the milk in a small saucepan, and heat until very warm (125°F to 130°F). Add the milk to the flour mixture, and stir for 1 minute. Stir in the egg white.

4. Add 2 tablespoons of the whole wheat flour to the dough, and stir to mix. Continue to add the flour in 2-tablespoon portions until a stiff dough is formed.

5. Sprinkle 2 tablespoons of the remaining whole wheat flour onto a flat surface, and turn the dough onto the surface. Knead the dough for 5 minutes, gradually adding enough of the remaining flour to form a smooth, satiny ball of dough.

6. Scrape the work surface, and lightly sprinkle it with flour. Return the dough to the surface, and, using a rolling pin, roll it into a 11-x-16-inch rectangle. Spread the cooled filling over the dough to within ½ inch of the edges, and roll the rectangle up jelly-roll style, beginning at the long end.

7. Coat a 12-inch round pizza pan or large baking sheet with nonstick cooking spray, and place the roll on the pan, bringing the ends together to form a ring. Using scissors, cut almost all of the way through the dough at 1-inch intervals. Twist each 1-inch segment to turn the cut side up. Cover the pan with a clean kitchen towel, and let rise in a warm place for about 35 minutes, or until doubled in size.

8. Lightly brush the top of the loaf with the skim milk or beaten egg white, and bake at 350°F for 16 to 18 minutes, or until lightly browned. Remove from the oven and let sit for 3 to 5 minutes.

9. To make the glaze, combine the glaze ingredients in a small bowl, stirring until smooth. Drizzle the glaze over the warm bread, and serve immediately.

Time-Saving Tip

To make the dough for Prune-Filled Tea Bread in a bread machine, simply place all of the dough ingredients in the machine's bread pan. (Do not heat the liquids.) Turn the machine to the "rise," "dough," "manual," or an equivalent setting so that the machine will mix, knead, and let the dough rise once. Check the dough about 5 minutes after the machine has started. If the dough seems too sticky, add more flour, a tablespoon at a time. If it seems too stiff, add more liquid, a teaspoon at a time. When the dough is ready, remove it from the machine and proceed to shape and bake it as directed in the recipe.

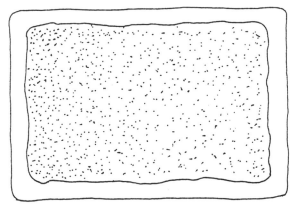

a. Spread the filling over the dough.

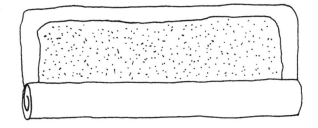

b. Roll the dough up jelly-roll style.

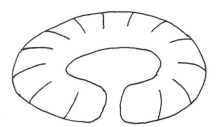

c. Bend the roll into a ring, and cut almost all the way through at 1-inch intervals.

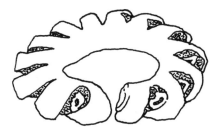

d. Twist each 1-inch segment to turn the cut side up.

Making Prune-Filled Tea Bread.

Applesauce Sticky Buns

Yield: 12 buns

DOUGH

1½ cups unbleached flour

2 tablespoons sugar

1½ teaspoons Rapid Rise yeast

¼ teaspoon salt

¾ cup plus 2 tablespoons
    unsweetened applesauce

1 egg white

¾ cup whole wheat flour

FILLING

2 tablespoons maple syrup

¼ teaspoon ground cinnamon

¼ cup plus 2 tablespoons dark raisins

3 tablespoons chopped walnuts
    (optional)

GLAZE

⅓ cup maple syrup

NUTRITIONAL FACTS (PER BUN)

Calories: 143	Fiber: 1.8 g
Chol: 0 mg	Protein: 3.1 g
Fat: 0.3 g	Sodium: 52 mg

---

1. To make the dough, combine the unbleached flour, sugar, yeast, and salt, and stir to mix well. Set aside.

2. Place the applesauce in a small saucepan, and heat until very warm (125°F to 130°F). Add the applesauce to the flour mixture, and stir for 1 minute. Stir in the egg white.

3. Add 2 tablespoons of the whole wheat flour to the dough, and stir to mix. Continue to add the flour in 2-tablespoon portions until a stiff dough is formed.

4. Sprinkle 2 tablespoons of the remaining whole wheat flour onto a flat surface, and turn the dough onto the surface. Knead the dough for 5 minutes, gradually adding enough of the remaining flour to form a smooth, satiny ball of dough.

5. Scrape the work surface, and lightly sprinkle it with flour. Return the dough to the surface, and, using a rolling pin, roll it into a 10-x-12-inch rectangle. Combine the 2 tablespoons of maple syrup and the cinnamon, and spread the mixture over the dough to within ½ inch of the edges. Sprinkle the raisins and, if desired, the walnuts over the syrup, and roll the rectangle up jelly-roll style, beginning at the long end.

6. Coat a 9-inch round pan with nonstick cooking spray, and pour the ⅓ cup of maple syrup over the bottom of the pan. Cut the rolled-up dough into 1-inch slices, and lay the slices in the pan, cut side up, spacing them ½ inch apart. Cover the pan with a clean kitchen towel, and let rise in a warm place for about 35 minutes, or until doubled in size.

7. Bake at 350°F for 20 minutes, or until lightly browned. Remove the pan from the oven, and run a knife around the edge of the pan to loosen the buns. Immediately invert the buns onto a serving plate, and serve warm.

Time-Saving Tip

Like the dough for the Prune-Filled Tea Bread, the dough for Applesauce Sticky Buns may be mixed in a bread machine. Just follow the directions on page 47.

Whole Wheat Apricot Bread

1. Combine the flour, sugar, baking powder, and baking soda in a large bowl, and stir to mix well. Set aside.

2. Drain the apricots, reserving the juice. Place the apricots in a blender, and process until smooth. Add enough of the reserved juice to bring the volume of the mixture up to 1½ cups.

3. Add the blended apricots and vanilla extract to the flour mixture, and stir just until the dry ingredients are moistened. Fold in the dried apricots and cereal.

4. Coat an 8-x-4-inch loaf pan with nonstick cooking spray. Spread the batter evenly in the pan, and bake at 325°F for 45 minutes, or just until a wooden toothpick inserted in the center of the loaf comes out clean.

5. Remove the bread from the oven, and let sit for 10 minutes. Turn the loaf onto a wire rack, and cool before slicing.

Yield: 16 slices

2 cups whole wheat flour

⅓ cup sugar

1 teaspoon baking powder

1 teaspoon baking soda

1 can (1 pound) apricots in juice, undrained

1 teaspoon vanilla extract

⅓ cup finely chopped dried apricots

⅓ cup barley nugget cereal or chopped pecans

NUTRITIONAL FACTS (PER SLICE)		
Calories: 94	Fat: 0.3 g	Protein: 2.6 g
Cholesterol: 0 mg	Fiber: 2.5 g	Sodium: 119 mg

4. Hors D'Oeuvres With a Difference

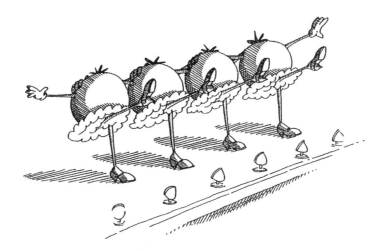

Food and festivity are part of the American way. Let's face it—great food really does liven up a party. Who can resist those creamy dips, those saucy meatballs, or those savory canapés? Unfortunately, traditional party favorites top the list of foods high in fat, sugar, and salt—ingredients that must be limited in a healthy diet. Fatty dips, spreads, meats, cheeses, crackers, and chips are often featured fare on hors d'oeuvres tables. Have a sample of each, and you could easily consume a full day's worth of fat and calories in an hour or two!

Enter low- and no-fat cheeses, nonfat sour cream, light mayonnaise, ultra-lean ground meats, reduced-fat lunch meats, and a host of other products that can help take the fat out of celebrations and get-togethers. You will be delighted to learn how a few simple ingredient substitutions can make a big fat difference in traditional party favorites. For instance, a bowl of dip made with a cup of full-fat sour cream gets about 500 calories and 48 grams of fat from the sour cream alone. Prepare the same dip with nonfat sour cream, and you will eliminate 320 calories and all 48 grams of fat. Scoop up your dip with some low-fat whole grain crackers—or, better yet, with raw carrot and celery sticks—and you will have a wholesome snack that is every bit as tempting as its full-fat counterpart.

This chapter presents a wide range of hot and cold hors d'oeuvres, both plain and fancy. From Shrimp Brushchetta to Fiesta Roll-Ups to Zippy Artichoke Dip, you will find a wealth of festive, party-perfect foods. Add some trays of fresh vegetables, a selection of in-season fruit, and plenty of low-cal beverages, and your menu will be high on satisfaction, yet remarkably low in fat. Friends and family will appreciate this more than you know.

Shrimp Bruschetta

Yield: 48 appetizers

6 ounces (about 1 cup) diced cooked shrimp

1 cup shredded nonfat or reduced-fat mozzarella cheese

$\frac{3}{4}$ cup chopped plum tomatoes (about $2\frac{1}{2}$ medium)

$\frac{3}{4}$ cup chopped fresh spinach

$\frac{1}{4}$ cup chopped scallions

1 teaspoon crushed fresh garlic

1 teaspoon dried oregano

1 long, thin loaf French bread (about 24 x 2 x 1 inches)

1. Combine the shrimp, cheese, tomatoes, spinach, scallions, garlic, and oregano in a medium-sized bowl, and stir to mix well. Set aside.

2. Slice the bread into 48 ($\frac{1}{2}$-inch) slices. Arrange the slices on a baking sheet, and bake at 300°F for 12 to 15 minutes, or until crisp and dry.

3. Spread each slice with 1 tablespoon of the shrimp mixture. Increase the oven temperature to 400°F, and return the appetizers to the oven for 5 minutes, or just until the cheese is melted.

4. Arrange the appetizers on a serving platter, and serve hot.

NUTRITIONAL FACTS (PER APPETIZER)		
Calories: 11	Fat: 0.1 g	Protein: 2 g
Cholesterol: 7 mg	Fiber: 0.2 g	Sodium: 54 mg

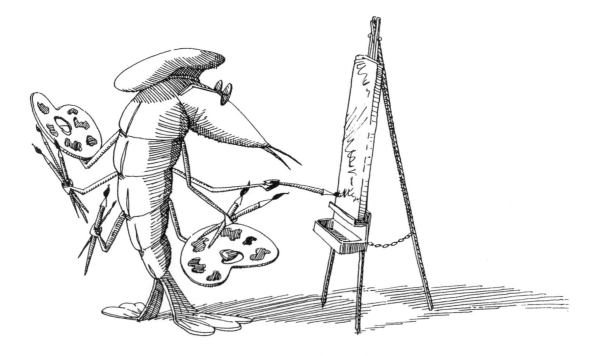

Crab-Stuffed Mushrooms

1. Remove and discard the mushroom stems. Wash the mushroom caps and pat dry. Set aside.

2. Combine the bread crumbs, crab meat, cheese, bell peppers, scallions, thyme, and black pepper in a medium-sized bowl, and stir to mix well. Add the egg whites and mayonnaise or sour cream, and stir gently to blend.

3. Coat a shallow baking pan with nonstick cooking spray. Place a heaping teaspoonful of stuffing in each mushroom cap, and arrange the mushrooms in the prepared pan.

4. Bake at 400°F for 20 minutes, or until lightly browned on top. Transfer the mushrooms to a serving platter, garnish with the lemon wedges, and serve hot.

Yield: 40 appetizers

40 medium-large fresh mushrooms

2 cups soft bread crumbs

8 ounces (1½ cups) finely flaked cooked crab meat

⅓ cup grated nonfat or reduced-fat Parmesan cheese

⅓ cup finely chopped red bell pepper

⅓ cup finely chopped green bell pepper

¼ cup finely chopped scallions

½ teaspoon dried thyme

¼ teaspoon ground black pepper

2 egg whites, lightly beaten

¼ cup nonfat mayonnaise or nonfat sour cream

Lemon wedges (garnish)

NUTRITIONAL FACTS (PER APPETIZER)

Calories: 19	Fat: 0.2 g	Protein: 1.9 g
Cholesterol: 4 mg	Fiber: 0.2 g	Sodium: 50 mg

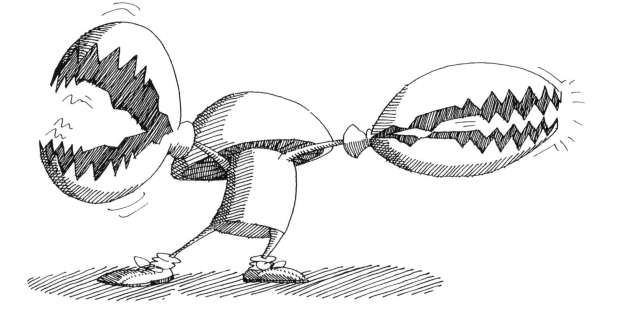

Aloha Meatballs

Yield: 45 appetizers

MEATBALLS

1 pound ground turkey breast or 96% lean ground beef

1 cup cooked brown rice

1 can (8 ounces) crushed pineapple in juice, drained

1 can (8 ounces) sliced water chestnuts, drained

½ cup chopped scallions

1 tablespoon reduced-sodium soy sauce

1 teaspoon ground ginger

SAUCE

¾ cup unsalted chicken broth

⅓ cup ketchup or chili sauce

3 tablespoons seasoned rice vinegar

2 tablespoons brown sugar

2 teaspoons cornstarch

½ teaspoon ground ginger

1. Combine the meatball ingredients in a medium-sized bowl, and mix thoroughly. Coat a baking sheet with nonstick cooking spray. Shape the meatball mixture into 45 (1-inch) balls, and place the meatballs on the baking sheet.

2. Bake at 350°F for about 25 minutes, or until thoroughly cooked. Transfer the meatballs to a chafing dish or Crock-Pot heated casserole to keep warm.

3. Combine the sauce ingredients in a small saucepan, and stir until the cornstarch is dissolved. Place over medium heat, and cook and stir until the mixture comes to a boil. Reduce the heat to low, and cook and stir for another minute, or until the mixture thickens slightly. Pour the sauce over the meatballs, toss gently to mix, and serve.

NUTRITIONAL FACTS (PER APPETIZER)

Calories: 24	Fat: 0.1 g	Protein: 2.5 g
Cholesterol: 6 mg	Fiber: 0.2 g	Sodium: 49 mg

Time-Saving Tip

To avoid a last-minute rush, make the meatballs in advance. Just cook them as directed—without the sauce—and freeze them in freezer bags. The day before the party, thaw the meatballs in the refrigerator. The next day, simply make the sauce and heat it along with the meatballs.

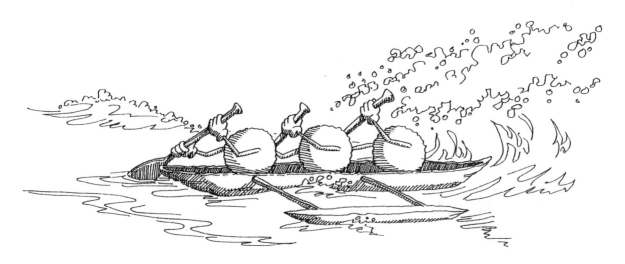

Chicken Fingers
With Honey Mustard Sauce

1. Place the corn flakes in a blender or food processor, and process into crumbs. (You should get about $^3/_4$ cup of crumbs. Adjust the amount if necessary.)

2. Combine the corn flake crumbs, poultry seasoning, and pepper in a shallow dish. Stir to mix well, and set aside.

3. Combine the egg substitute and milk in a shallow dish. Stir to mix well, and set aside.

4. Cut each chicken breast half into 5 long strips. Dip each strip first in the egg mixture, and then in the crumb mixture, turning to coat each side with crumbs.

5. Coat a large baking sheet with nonstick cooking spray, and arrange the strips in a single layer on the sheet. Spray the tops of the strips lightly with cooking spray, and bake at 400°F for 15 minutes, or until the strips are golden brown and no longer pink inside.

6. While the chicken is baking, combine the sauce ingredients in a small dish, and stir to mix well. Arrange the chicken strips on a serving platter, and serve hot, accompanied by the bowl of sauce.

Yield: 20 appetizers

3 cups corn flakes

$^1/_2$ teaspoon poultry seasoning

$^1/_4$ teaspoon ground black pepper

3 tablespoons fat-free egg substitute

3 tablespoons skim milk

1 pound boneless skinless chicken breasts (about 4 breast halves)

Nonstick cooking spray

SAUCE

$^1/_4$ cup plus 2 tablespoons nonfat or reduced-fat mayonnaise

3 tablespoons spicy mustard

3 tablespoons honey

2 tablespoons lemon juice

NUTRITIONAL FACTS
(PER APPETIZER, WITH 2 TEASPOONS OF SAUCE)

Calories: 51	Fat: 0.4 g	Protein: 5.8 g
Cholesterol: 13 mg	Fiber: 0.1 g	Sodium: 111 mg

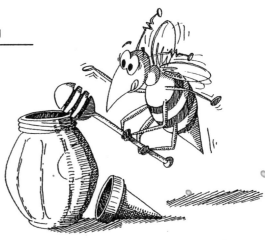

Stuffed Finger Sandwiches

Yield: 18 appetizers

1 long, thin loaf French bread (about 24 x 2 x 1 inches)

½ cup plus 2 tablespoons nonfat cream cheese

½ teaspoon dried Italian seasoning

¾ teaspoon crushed fresh garlic

4 ounces thinly sliced cooked turkey breast

8–10 fresh tender spinach leaves

½ medium red bell pepper, cut in thin strips

½ cup chopped frozen (thawed) artichoke hearts, or ½ cup drained and chopped canned artichoke hearts

1. Using a serrated knife, slice the French bread lengthwise, cutting off the top third of the loaf. Using your fingers, remove and discard enough of the soft inner bread to leave only a ½-inch-thick shell.

2. Combine the cream cheese, Italian seasoning, and garlic in a small bowl, and stir to mix well. Spread half of this mixture evenly over the inside of the bottom shell. Roll up the turkey slices, and arrange them in an even layer over the cream cheese mixture. Lay the spinach leaves over the turkey, and top with a layer of pepper strips. Finish with a layer of artichokes.

3. Spread the remaining cream cheese mixture over the inside of the top shell. Place the top shell over the bottom shell to reform the loaf, and wrap the loaf tightly in aluminum foil or plastic wrap. Chill for several hours or overnight.

4. When ready to serve, unwrap the loaf, and use a serrated knife to cut the loaf diagonally into 1-inch slices. Secure each piece with a wooden toothpick, arrange on a platter, and serve.

NUTRITIONAL FACTS (PER APPETIZER)		
Calories: 60	Fat: 0.2 g	Protein: 5.5 g
Cholesterol: 8 mg	Fiber: 0.7 g	Sodium: 179 mg

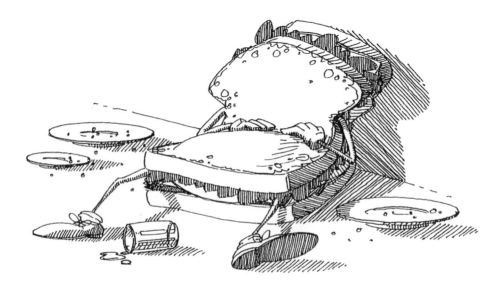

Fiesta Roll-Ups

1. Combine the sour cream and picante sauce in a small bowl. Stir to mix, and set aside.

2. Spread each tortilla with 3 tablespoons of cream cheese, extending the cheese to the outer edges. Lay 2 ounces of sliced turkey or ham over the *bottom half only* of each tortilla, leaving a 1-inch margin on each outer edge. Place 1 ounce of Cheddar over the turkey, and spread with 1 tablespoon of the sour cream-picante mixture. Arrange 1 lettuce leaf over the cheese, and sprinkle with 1 tablespoon of olives. Arrange 3 tomato slices over the olive layer, and top with 2 tablespoons of scallions.

3. Starting at the bottom, roll each tortilla up tightly. Cut a $1\frac{1}{4}$-inch piece off each end, and discard. Slice the remainder of each tortilla into six $1\frac{1}{4}$-inch pieces. Arrange the rolls on a platter, and serve.

Yield: 48 appetizers

$\frac{1}{4}$ cup nonfat sour cream

$\frac{1}{4}$ cup picante sauce

8 fat-free flour tortillas (10-inch rounds)

$1\frac{1}{2}$ cups nonfat or reduced-fat cream cheese

1 pound thinly sliced cooked turkey breast, or 1 pound thinly sliced ham (at least 97% lean)

8 ounces thinly sliced nonfat or reduced-fat Cheddar cheese

8 large fresh lettuce leaves

$\frac{1}{2}$ cup chopped black olives

24 very thin slices of tomato

$\frac{1}{2}$ cup sliced scallions

NUTRITIONAL FACTS (PER APPETIZER)

Calories: 48	Fat: 0.2 g	Protein: 5.8 g
Cholesterol: 9 mg	Fiber: 0.3 g	Sodium: 136 mg

Time-Saving Tip

To avoid a last-minute rush, make Fiesta Roll-Ups the day before your party, cover the hors d'oeuvres with plastic wrap, and refrigerate. When guests arrive, simply remove the plastic wrap and serve.

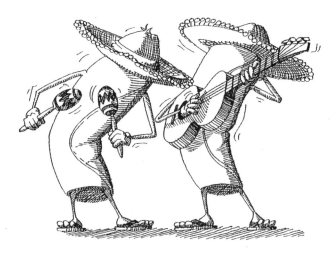

Mexican Bean Dip

Yield: 2½ cups

1 can (1 pound) pinto beans, rinsed and drained

¼ cup nonfat sour cream

2–3 teaspoons chili powder

½ teaspoon ground cumin

½ cup shredded nonfat or reduced-fat Cheddar cheese

¼ cup thinly sliced scallions

¼ cup sliced black olives

2 tablespoons finely chopped jalapeño peppers

1. Place the beans, sour cream, chili powder, and cumin in a food processor or blender, and process until smooth. Spread the mixture over the bottom of a 9-inch glass pie pan. Top with the cheese, followed by the scallions, olives, and jalapeños.

2. Serve at room temperature or hot. If using a microwave oven, heat at high power for 5 to 6 minutes, or until the edges are bubbly and the cheese is melted. If using a conventional oven, bake at 400°F for 20 minutes. Serve with fat-free tortilla chips.

NUTRITIONAL FACTS (PER TABLESPOON)		
Calories: 14	Fat: 0.1 g	Protein: 1.2 g
Cholesterol: 0 mg	Fiber: 0.7 g	Sodium: 44 mg

Blender Salsa

Yield: 2¼ cups

1 can (1 pound) unsalted whole tomatoes, undrained

½ cup chopped onion

1–2 tablespoons chopped jalapeño peppers

1–2 tablespoons minced fresh cilantro

2 tablespoons red wine vinegar

1 teaspoon chili powder

½ teaspoon salt

This easy-to-make salsa has 75 percent less sodium than most bottled brands.

1. Place all of the ingredients in a food processor or blender, and blend for 5 to 10 seconds, or until well mixed but slightly chunky. Transfer the salsa to a serving dish, cover, and chill for several hours to blend the flavors.

2. Serve with fat-free tortilla chips.

NUTRITIONAL FACTS (PER TABLESPOON)		
Calories: 4	Fat: 0 g	Protein: 0.2 g
Cholesterol: 0 mg	Fiber: 0.3 g	Sodium: 35 mg

Zippy Artichoke Dip

1. Combine the sour cream, mayonnaise, mustard, garlic, and pepper in a medium-sized bowl, and stir to mix well. Stir in the artichokes. Transfer the dip to a serving dish, cover, and chill for several hours.

2. Serve with whole grain crackers and raw vegetables.

Yield: 2¼ cups

1 cup nonfat sour cream

½ cup nonfat or reduced-fat mayonnaise

1 tablespoon grainy Dijon mustard

½ teaspoon crushed fresh garlic

¼ teaspoon coarsely ground black pepper

1 can (14 ounces) artichoke hearts, well drained and chopped

NUTRITIONAL FACTS (PER TABLESPOON)
Calories: 9	Fat: 0 g	Protein: 0.7 g
Cholesterol: 0 mg	Fiber: 0.4 g	Sodium: 51 mg

Hot and Creamy Crab Dip

1. Cut the top from the bread loaf, and set aside. Hollow out the bread, leaving a 1-inch-thick shell. Set aside.

2. Coat a baking sheet with nonstick cooking spray. Cut the removed bread into cubes, and place on the baking sheet. Bake at 350°F for 10 minutes, or until lightly toasted. Set aside.

3. Place the cream cheese, milk, lemon juice, and Worcestershire sauce in a food processor, and process until smooth. Stir in the crab meat and onion. Evenly spread the mixture in the hollowed loaf, cover with the bread top, and wrap in aluminum foil.

4. Bake the filled loaf at 350°F for 1 hour and 15 minutes, or until the dip is hot and creamy. Place the loaf on a serving plate, remove and discard the top, and sprinkle the dip lightly with paprika. Serve hot with whole grain crackers and the toasted bread cubes.

Yield: 3¼ cups

1 large round loaf sourdough bread

2 cups nonfat or reduced-fat cream cheese, softened

2 tablespoons skim milk

1 tablespoon lemon juice

1 tablespoon white wine Worcestershire sauce

1½ cups (about 8 ounces) flaked cooked crab meat

2 tablespoons finely chopped onion

Ground paprika

NUTRITIONAL FACTS (PER TABLESPOON)
Calories: 13	Fat: 0.1 g	Protein: 2.2 g
Cholesterol: 4 mg	Fiber: 0 g	Sodium: 61 mg

Nut 'n' Honey Dip

Yield: 2¼ cups

2 cups nonfat ricotta cheese

¼ cup honey

3–4 tablespoons smooth or chunky peanut butter

1. Place all of the ingredients in a food processor or blender, and process until well blended. Transfer the dip to a serving dish, cover, and chill for several hours.

2. Serve with sliced apples and pears, chunks of banana, whole fresh strawberries, and fresh pineapple spears.

NUTRITIONAL FACTS (PER TABLESPOON)

Calories: 23	Fat: 0.6 g	Protein: 2 g
Cholesterol: 1 mg	Fiber: 0 g	Sodium: 29 mg

Commendable Crackers and Chips

One of the most healthful and satisfying complements to a tempting dip or spread is a bowl of low-fat whole grain crackers and chips. The list below includes just some of the lowest-fat brands now available in your grocery and health foods stores. When heartier accompaniments are desired, try thinly sliced rounds of whole grain bagels; fingers of firm whole wheat, rye, or pumpernickel bread; or wedges of toasted whole grain pita. These snacks are so delicious that you will find yourself serving them not just at party time, but whenever you're in the mood for a light and healthy snack.

Crackers	**Crackers**	**Chips**
Finn Crisp	Pepperidge Farm	Baked Tostitos
Hain Fat-Free	Wholesome Choice	Guiltless Gourmet Fat-Free
Harvest Crisps	Ry Vita	Tortilla Chips
Health Valley	Rye Krisp	Louise's Fat-Free and
Hol Grain	Stoned Wheat Thins	Reduced-Fat Potato Chips
Kavli Norwegian Flatbread	Triscuits (reduced fat)	Louise's Reduced-Fat
Krispy Cakes	Wasa Bread	Tortilla Chips
Melba Toast	Wheat Thins (reduced fat)	Smart Temptations
Mini Rice Cakes		Tortilla Chips

Dilly Cucumber Dip

1. Place the cucumber in a food processor or blender, and process until finely chopped. Roll the cucumber in a clean kitchen towel, and squeeze out any excess moisture.

2. Combine the sour cream and mayonnaise in a medium-sized bowl, and fold in the cucumber and all of the remaining ingredients. Transfer the dip to a serving dish, cover, and chill for several hours.

3. Serve with raw vegetables, whole grain crackers, chunks of pumpernickel or sourdough bread, and smoked salmon.

Yield: 2¼ cups

1 medium cucumber, peeled, seeded, and cut into chunks

1½ cups nonfat sour cream

½ cup nonfat or reduced-fat mayonnaise

2 tablespoons finely chopped onion

1 tablespoon plus 1½ teaspoons finely chopped fresh dill

NUTRITIONAL FACTS (PER TABLESPOON)

Calories: 13	Fat: 0 g	Protein: 0.4 g
Cholesterol: 0 mg	Fiber: 0 g	Sodium: 41 mg

Bacon and Cheddar Dip

1. Place the cream cheese, sour cream, and mayonnaise in a food processor, and process to mix well. Stir in the Cheddar cheese, bacon, and onion. Transfer the dip to a serving dish, cover, and chill for several hours.

2. Serve with whole grain crackers and raw vegetables.

Yield: 3 cups

1 cup nonfat cream cheese, softened

1 cup nonfat sour cream

½ cup nonfat or reduced-fat mayonnaise

1 cup shredded nonfat or reduced-fat Cheddar cheese

4 slices turkey bacon, cooked, drained, and crumbled

2 tablespoons plus 1½ teaspoons finely chopped onion

NUTRITIONAL FACTS (PER TABLESPOON)

Calories: 17	Fat: 0.2 g	Protein: 1.8 g
Cholesterol: 2 mg	Fiber: 0 g	Sodium: 80 mg

5. Soups That Satisfy

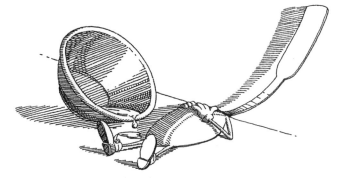

There's nothing quite as warming and comforting as a steaming bowl of homemade soup. And soups are naturals for fat-free and low-fat cooking. Lean meats and poultry, whole grains, pasta, beans, and vegetables can be combined to produce a variety of culinary creations that are satisfying without being fattening.

Watching your weight? Soups can help. Soups take longer to eat than most foods, so that less food and fewer calories are consumed in the twenty-minute period it takes for the brain to realize that the stomach is full. This helps prevent overeating.

Soups are perhaps the most versatile of foods, and so are as much a boon to the menu planner as they are to the calorie counter. A light soup is the perfect introduction to a full meal. A more substantial soup needs only crusty whole grain bread and perhaps a salad to make a satisfying lunch or light supper. Grabbing your lunches away from home? Take along a thermos of hot soup, and you'll have a nourishing meal on hand whenever you get hungry.

Even when you take the time to make soups from scratch, you'll find that soups are perfect for a busy lifestyle. Most soups can be prepared whenever you have the time, and then refrigerated or frozen until needed. In fact, many taste even better when refrigerated overnight, allowing the flavors to marry and blend.

Of course, homemade soups have more than one advantage over commercial brews. Made from fresh, wholesome ingredients, homemade soups are bursting with nutrients and garden-fresh flavor. Just as important, while most commercially prepared soups are loaded with fat and salt, your soups can easily be made low in sodium and, of course, practically fat-free. Will your low-salt soups taste flat? Absolutely not! Herbs like oregano, marjoram, and thyme; a dash of sherry; a clove or two of garlic; and other flavorful ingredients will make your soups so savory, no one will miss the salt.

This chapter presents a variety of delectable low-fat, low-salt soups. Whether you are looking for a golden broth floating with tender noodles and chunks of turkey or a thick and creamy chowder, there's a soup that will meet your needs deliciously. You'll even find tips for giving your favorite soup recipe a slimming makeover. So take out your kettle, and get ready to make soups a healthful part of your menus.

Pasta Fagioli Soup

Yield: 12 servings

1 pound 96% lean ground beef or ground turkey breast

1 large onion, chopped

1 large carrot, peeled, halved, and sliced

2 large stalks celery with leaves, thinly sliced

2 cans (1 pound each) unsalted tomatoes, crushed

1 teaspoon dried basil

1 teaspoon dried oregano

1 teaspoon crushed fresh garlic

¼ teaspoon ground black pepper

3 cups beef broth

1 can (1 pound) navy or garbanzo beans, rinsed and drained

6 ounces elbow macaroni or ziti pasta

1. Place the ground meat in a 4-quart pot, and brown over medium heat, stirring constantly to crumble, until the meat is no longer pink. Drain off any excess fat. (If the meat is 96-percent lean, there should be no fat.)

2. Add the onion, carrot, celery, tomatoes, seasonings, and beef broth to the pot, and bring to a boil over high heat. Reduce the heat to low, cover, and simmer for 15 minutes, or until the vegetables are tender.

3. Add the beans and pasta to the pot, cover, and simmer for 7 to 9 minutes, or just until the pasta is al dente. (Be careful not to overcook, as the pasta will continue to soften as long as it remains in the hot soup.)

4. Ladle the soup into individual serving bowls, and serve hot.

NUTRITIONAL FACTS (PER 1-CUP SERVING)		
Calories: 152	Fat: 2 g	Protein: 12.2 g
Cholesterol: 18 mg	Fiber: 3.5 g	Sodium: 363 mg

Turkey Barley Soup

Yield: 8 servings

6 cups unsalted chicken broth or water

¾ cup hulled barley

2 cups sliced fresh mushrooms

1 cup sliced carrots

1 cup sliced celery (include leaves)

1 cup chopped onion

2 teaspoons chicken bouillon granules

1 teaspoon dried thyme

¼ teaspoon ground black pepper

2 cups diced cooked turkey breast

1. Combine the broth or water and the barley in a 3-quart pot, and bring to a boil over high heat. Reduce the heat to low, cover, and simmer for 40 minutes, or until the barley is almost tender.

2. Add the mushrooms, carrots, celery, onion, bouillon granules, thyme, pepper, and turkey to the pot. Cover and simmer for 20 minutes, or until the barley and vegetables are tender.

3. Ladle the soup into individual serving bowls, and serve hot.

NUTRITIONAL FACTS (PER 1-CUP SERVING)		
Calories: 135	Fat: 0.9 g	Protein: 13 g
Cholesterol: 30 mg	Fiber: 3.5 g	Sodium: 285 mg

Golden Turkey Noodle Soup

1. Combine the broth or water, sweet potatoes, onion, bouillon granules, and pepper in a 3-quart pot, and bring to a boil over high heat. Reduce the heat to low, cover, and simmer for 15 ~~es, or until the potatoes are tender.~~

~~move the pot from the heat. Using a slotted spoon, transfer weet potatoes to a blender. Add 1½ cups of the hot broth to blender, and place the lid on the blender, leaving the top ntly ajar to allow steam to escape. Carefully blend the mixture low speed until smooth.~~

3. Return the blended mixture to the pot, and place over high heat. Add the carrots and celery, and bring the mixture to a boil. Reduce the heat to low, cover, and simmer for 6 to 8 minutes, or until the vegetables are barely tender.

4. Add the noodles and turkey or chicken to the pot, cover, and simmer, stirring occasionally, for about 8 minutes, or just until the noodles are al dente. (Be careful not to overcook, as the pasta will continue to soften as long as it remains in the hot soup.)

5. Ladle the soup into individual serving bowls, and serve hot.

Yield: 8 servings

6½ cups unsalted chicken broth or water

1½ cups diced peeled sweet potatoes (about 1½ medium)

1 medium onion, chopped

2 teaspoons chicken bouillon granules

⅛ teaspoon ground white pepper

1 medium carrot, peeled and diced

1 stalk celery with leaves, thinly sliced

4 ounces medium no-yolk noodles

2 cups diced cooked turkey breast or chicken breast

NUTRITIONAL FACTS (PER 1-CUP SERVING)

Calories: 151	Fat: 0.9 g	Protein: 13 g
Cholesterol: 30 mg	Fiber: 1.7 g	Sodium: 287 mg

Barley and Cheese Soup

Yield: 6 servings

2 cups water

½ teaspoon chicken bouillon granules

½ cup plus 1 tablespoon
quick-cooking barley

2 tablespoons finely chopped onion

3 cups skim milk, divided

2 tablespoons cornstarch

⅓ cup instant nonfat dry milk powder

⅛ teaspoon cayenne pepper or
ground white pepper

1 cup shredded nonfat processed
Cheddar cheese, or 1 cup shredded
reduced-fat Cheddar cheese

3 tablespoons thinly sliced scallions
(garnish)

1. Combine the water, bouillon granules, barley, and onion in a 2½-quart pot, and bring to a boil over high heat. Reduce the heat to low, cover, and simmer for 10 to 12 minutes, or until the barley is tender.

2. Combine ¼ cup of the milk and all of the cornstarch in a small bowl, and stir until the cornstarch dissolves. Set aside.

3. In a medium-sized bowl, combine the remaining 2¾ cups of milk with the milk powder and the cayenne or white pepper, and mix until smooth. Add the milk to the pot, increase the heat to medium, and cook, stirring constantly, just until the mixture begins to boil.

4. Stir the cornstarch mixture once, and add it to the pot. Cook and stir for 1 minute, or until the mixture thickens slightly.

5. Add the cheese to the pot, and stir until the cheese melts. Remove the pot from the heat, ladle the soup into individual serving bowls, and garnish each serving with a sprinkling of scallions. Serve hot.

NUTRITIONAL FACTS (PER 1-CUP SERVING)		
Calories: 145	Fat: 0.5 g	Protein: 13 g
Cholesterol: 6 mg	Fiber: 1.6 g	Sodium: 316 mg

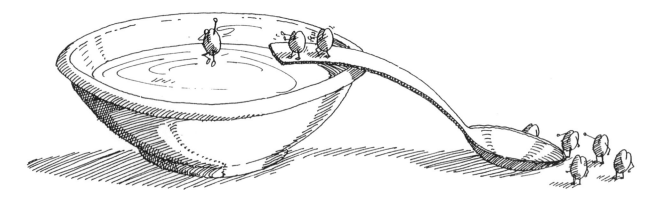

Fresh Corn Chowder

1. Combine the water, potatoes, celery, onion, bouillon granules, savory, and pepper in a 3-quart pot, and bring to a boil over high heat. Reduce the heat to low, cover, and simmer for 15 minutes, or until the potatoes are almost tender.

2. Add the corn to the pot. Cover and simmer for 5 minutes, or until the potatoes and corn are tender.

3. Place the milk in a medium-sized bowl, and stir in the milk powder. Add the mixture to the pot, and cook, stirring constantly, for about 5 minutes, or until the mixture is heated through.

4. Remove 4 cups of soup—including both broth and vegetables—from the pot. Place 2 cups of the removed soup in a blender, and place the lid on the blender, leaving the top slightly ajar to allow steam to escape. Carefully blend the mixture at low speed until smooth. Return the blended mixture to the pot, and repeat this procedure with the remaining 2 cups of soup.

5. Simmer the soup for 5 additional minutes. Ladle the soup into individual serving bowls, and garnish each serving with a sprinkling of chives or scallions. Serve hot.

Yield: 9 servings

1 cup water

4 cups diced peeled potatoes (about 1½ pounds)

½ cup thinly sliced celery

½ cup chopped onion

2½ teaspoons chicken bouillon granules

1½ teaspoons dried savory

¼ teaspoon ground white pepper

4 cups fresh or frozen (thawed) whole kernel corn (about 1½ pounds)

3 cups skim milk

¼ cup plus 2 tablespoons instant nonfat dry milk powder

3 tablespoons finely chopped fresh chives or scallions (garnish)

NUTRITIONAL FACTS (PER 1-CUP SERVING)		
Calories: 164	Fat: 1.1 g	Protein: 7.8 g
Cholesterol: 2 mg	Fiber: 3.1 g	Sodium: 360 mg

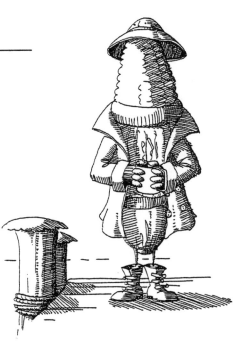

Getting the Fat Out of
Your Soup Recipes

Almost everyone has a favorite soup recipe or two. Maybe it's a recipe for Grandma's Chicken Noodle Soup—the one she always made for you when you were sick. Or maybe it's a recipe for the Split Pea With Ham Soup that always appears on your mother's holiday table. More than likely, though, your favorite soup recipe is a little high in fat—especially if it's a cream soup or if it contains meat. If the recipe uses a commercial broth, it may also be high in salt. Fortunately, it's easy to reduce fat and salt in just about any soup recipe you can think of. Here are some tips.

Reducing Fat

❑ If your recipe contains beef, pork, or poultry, use the leanest cuts available, and trim off any visible fats. (See Chapter 1 for a discussion of lean meats and poultry.) If you have to brown the meat before adding it to the soup, be sure to drain off any fat before placing the meat in the soup pot.

❑ After preparing a meat stock or soup, refrigerate it for a few hours or overnight to allow the fat to rise to the top and harden. Lift off the hardened fat for a fat-free broth that has almost no calories.

❑ When there's no time to refrigerate your stock or broth, defat it quickly by placing it in a fat separator cup. This specially designed cup has a spout that pours stock from the bottom of the cup. The fat, which floats to the top, stays in the cup.

❑ If you don't have a fat separator cup, quickly defat your soup with ice cubes. Just place a few ice cubes in a pot of warm—not hot—soup, and let the cubes remain in the stock for a few seconds. Then remove the cubes, as well as the fat that clings to them.

❑ If you choose to use a canned broth, keep in mind that most broths are quite low in fat, and that any fat that is present will have floated to the top. When you open the can, simply spoon out and discard the fat. Now you have a fat-free broth!

❑ If your recipe contains milk, substitute 1-percent low-fat or skim milk for the whole milk. For a richer taste, add one to two tablespoons of instant nonfat dry milk powder to each cup of low-fat or skim milk.

❑ If your recipe contains cream, substitute evaporated skim milk—or one cup of skim or low-fat milk mixed with one-third cup of instant nonfat dry milk powder—for the high-fat cream.

❑ To add extra richness to low-fat cream soups, purée some of the broth and vegetables from the soup. Then return the mixture to the pot to thicken the soup.

❑ If your recipe contains sour cream, substitute a reduced-fat or nonfat brand for the full-fat product.

❑ If your recipe contains cheese, use a reduced-fat or nonfat brand. Most reduced-fat cheeses melt well, although they should be finely shredded for best results. When using nonfat cheeses, always choose a processed cheese, which is specifically designed to melt during cooking.

Reducing Salt

❑ If your recipe has a stock or bouillon base, either use a commercial salt-free or low-salt stock, or make your own stock.

❒ To make your soup more flavorful without using salt, reduce your stock or broth by simmering it uncovered until some of the liquid evaporates. This will intensify the flavors.

❒ To prevent your low-salt soup from tasting flat, add a little lemon juice or vinegar to the finished product. These ingredients give the impression of saltiness.

❒ When decreasing the amount of salt or salty bouillon in a recipe, increase the herbs and spices for added flavor.

❒ Add a pinch of white pepper to your pot of low-salt soup. The pungency of the spice will reduce the need for salt.

Creamy Mushroom Soup

Yield: 5 servings

1. Combine the mushrooms, onions, sherry, marjoram or thyme, salt, and pepper in a $2\frac{1}{2}$-quart pot. Place over medium heat, and cook, stirring frequently, until the mushrooms are tender and most of the liquid has evaporated.

2. Add $2\frac{1}{2}$ cups of the milk and all of the evaporated skim milk to the pot. Cook and stir until the mixture comes to a simmer.

3. Combine the remaining $\frac{1}{2}$ cup of milk and the flour in a jar with a tight-fitting lid, and shake until smooth. Add the flour mixture to the soup, and cook and stir until thickened and bubbly.

4. Ladle the soup into individual serving bowls, and serve hot.

4 cups sliced fresh mushrooms

$\frac{1}{2}$ cup chopped onion

2 tablespoons dry sherry

1 teaspoon dried marjoram or thyme

$\frac{1}{2}$ teaspoon salt

$\frac{1}{8}$ teaspoon ground white pepper

3 cups skim milk, divided

1 cup evaporated skim milk

$\frac{1}{3}$ cup toasted garbanzo flour* or unbleached flour

NUTRITIONAL FACTS (PER 1-CUP SERVING)

Calories: 140	Fat: 0.9 g	Protein: 12 g
Cholesterol: 0 mg	Fiber: 1.9 g	Sodium: 330 mg

*An excellent thickener for soups, stews, and gravies, garbanzo flour is made by grinding toasted garbanzo beans. This wholesome flour adds a rich nutty flavor to dishes, and boosts nutritional value. Look for it in health foods stores and many grocery stores.

Summer Vegetable Soup

Yield: 7 servings

1½ pounds ripe tomatoes (about 4 medium), diced

2 cups unsalted vegetable broth or water

4 cups chopped cabbage

1 cup fresh or frozen (thawed) whole kernel corn

1 cup fresh or frozen (thawed) cut green beans

1 medium onion, chopped

1 medium carrot, peeled, halved, and sliced

¾ teaspoon salt

¼ teaspoon ground black pepper

1 teaspoon dried thyme or marjoram

¼ teaspoon celery seed

2 tablespoons tomato paste

1. Combine the tomatoes and the broth or water in a 4-quart pot, and bring to a boil over high heat. Reduce the heat to low, cover, and simmer for 20 minutes, or until the tomatoes are soft.

2. Add the remaining ingredients to the pot, and simmer for 15 minutes, or until the vegetables are tender.

3. Ladle the soup into individual serving bowls, and serve hot.

NUTRITIONAL FACTS (PER 1-CUP SERVING)

Calories: 68	Fat: 0.8 g	Protein: 2.9 g
Cholesterol: 0 mg	Fiber: 3.7 g	Sodium: 256 mg

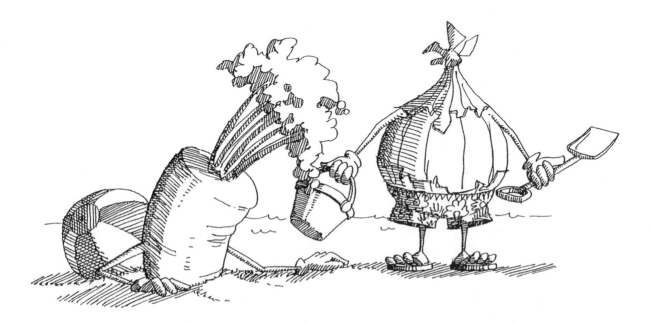

Tomato Florentine Soup *add some chicken*

Yield: 7 servings

1. Coat a 3-quart pot with cooking spray or olive oil, and place over medium heat. Add the onions, and sauté for 3 minutes, or until the onions are soft.

2. Add the tomatoes, vegetable broth or water, tomato paste, salt, pepper, and Italian seasoning to the pot. Increase the heat to high, and bring to a boil. Add the pasta, cover, and cook over medium-low heat for 8 minutes, or until the pasta is almost al dente.

3. Add the spinach to the pot, and simmer for 1 to 2 minutes, or just until the pasta is al dente and the spinach is wilted. (Be careful not to overcook, as the pasta will continue to soften as long as it remains in the hot soup.)

4. Ladle the soup into individual bowls, topping each serving with a tablespoon of cheese, if desired. Serve hot.

Olive oil cooking spray or 1 tablespoon olive oil

1 medium onion, chopped

1 can (1 pound) unsalted tomatoes, crushed

4 cups unsalted vegetable broth or water

2 tablespoons tomato paste

¾ teaspoon salt

¼ teaspoon ground black pepper

1 teaspoon dried Italian seasoning

4 ounces sea shell pasta

2 cups (packed) chopped fresh spinach

½ cup grated nonfat or reduced-fat Parmesan cheese (optional)

NUTRITIONAL FACTS (PER 1-CUP SERVING)		
Calories: 125	Fat: 0.7 g	Protein: 4.5 g
Cholesterol: 0 mg	Fiber: 3.4 g	Sodium: 258 mg

Golden Split Pea Soup

Yield: 8 servings

1. Combine all of the ingredients in a 3-quart pot, and bring to a boil over high heat. Reduce the heat to low, cover, and simmer, stirring occasionally, for 1 hour, or until the peas are soft and the liquid is thick.

2. Ladle the soup into individual serving bowls, and serve hot.

1½ cups dried yellow split peas, cleaned (page 148)

1 medium yellow onion, chopped

2 medium sweet potatoes, peeled and diced

6 cups unsalted chicken broth or water

2 teaspoons chicken bouillon granules

2 teaspoons ground cumin

2 teaspoons ground coriander

½ teaspoon ground ginger

½ teaspoon ground turmeric

⅛ teaspoon ground white pepper

NUTRITIONAL FACTS (PER 1-CUP SERVING)		
Calories: 177	Fat: 0.8 g	Protein: 10 g
Cholesterol: 0 mg	Fiber: 7 g	Sodium: 255 mg

Spanish Bean Soup

Yield: 9 servings

1¼ cups dried garbanzo beans, cleaned and soaked (page 148)

8 cups unsalted chicken broth or water

1 large Spanish onion, chopped

1 teaspoon crushed fresh garlic

6 ounces ham (at least 97% lean), diced, or 6 ounces smoked turkey sausage (at least 97% lean), diced

1¼ teaspoons chicken bouillon granules

¼ teaspoon ground white pepper

¾ pound unpeeled potatoes (about 2 medium), diced

1 teaspoon dried saffron

3 tablespoons finely chopped fresh parsley

1. Combine the beans and the chicken broth or water in a 4-quart pot, and bring to a boil over high heat. Reduce the heat to low, cover, and simmer, stirring occasionally, for 1½ to 2 hours, or until the beans are tender.

2. Add all of the remaining ingredients except for the parsley to the pot, cover, and simmer for about 30 minutes, or until the potatoes are tender.

3. Stir the parsley into the soup. Ladle the soup into individual serving bowls, and serve hot.

NUTRITIONAL FACTS (PER 1-CUP SERVING)		
Calories: 172	Fat: 2.3 g	Protein: 10 g
Cholesterol: 9 mg	Fiber: 4.8 g	Sodium: 327 mg

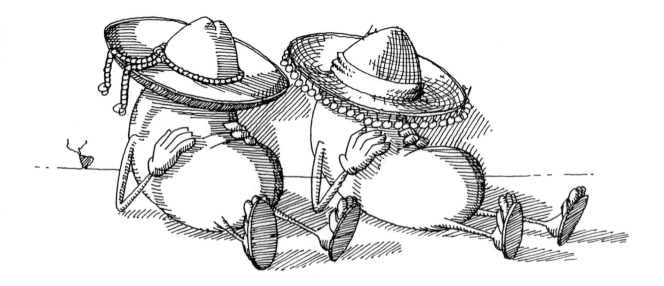

6. Well-Dressed Salads

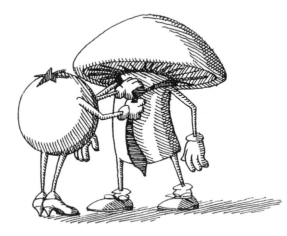

Everyone knows that salads are healthful—low in fat and calories, and high in fiber, vitamins, and minerals. Beware, though; a low-fat salad quickly becomes a nutritional disaster when high-fat cheeses and mayonnaise- or oil-based dressings are piled on.

Take the typical salad bar lunch, for instance. A pile of fresh, crisp greens makes for a good start. But then comes the shredded cheese, hard boiled eggs, fried croutons, and mayonnaise-laden potato or tuna salad, not to mention the dressing. A salad dressing ladle usually holds 2 tablespoons of dressing. For most dressings, this amounts to about 160 calories and 17 grams of fat! All things considered, it would be easy to walk away with 50 grams of fat on your plate.

Fortunately, when you make salads at home, you can control what goes into them. Ingredients like nonfat mayonnaise and nonfat sour cream make it possible to create fat-free versions of potato salad, cole slaw, and other family favor-

ites. Bottled nonfat salad dressings, nonfat cheeses, and ultra-lean lunch meats are also salad-making essentials. This chapter uses these ingredients plus plenty of fresh veggies, fruits, whole grains, beans, and pasta to make a variety of palate-pleasing creations. Need a dressing for your fresh-tossed salads that won't blow your fat and sodium budgets? This chapter presents a variety of tasty low- and no-fat dressings with just a fraction of the sodium of most commercial brands. You'll even find a recipe for crunchy low-fat croutons that will give your salad the perfect crowning touch.

So whether you're looking for a lighter way of dressing your favorite tossed green salad, a low-fat but luscious spin on potato salad, a cooling cucumber salad, or a show-stopping fruit salad, you need look no further. You'll find that any salad can be made delicious, satisfying, *and* healthy once you know the secrets of fat-free cooking.

Antipasto Salad

Yield: 8 servings

8 cups torn romaine lettuce

¾ cup shredded nonfat or reduced-fat mozzarella cheese

3 ounces thinly shaved turkey pastrami (at least 97% lean)

½ small red bell pepper, cut into thin rings

½ small green bell pepper, cut into thin rings

4 thin slices red onion, separated into rings

¾ cup canned garbanzo beans, rinsed and drained

8 cherry tomatoes, halved

8 Greek salad peppers

8 large pitted black olives (optional)

1. Arrange the lettuce over the bottom of a large serving platter, and sprinkle with the cheese. Cut the pastrami into thin strips, and arrange over the cheese. Spread the bell pepper and onion rings over the top.

2. Arrange the garbanzo beans, tomatoes, salad peppers, and olives, if desired, around the outer edges of the lettuce. Serve with a dish of bottled nonfat Italian dressing or Creamy Italian Dressing (page 78).

NUTRITIONAL FACTS (PER 1½-CUP SERVING)

Calories: 73	Fat: 0.9 g	Protein: 8 g
Cholesterol: 7 mg	Fiber: 2.1 g	Sodium: 244 mg

Spicy Beet Salad

Yield: 10 servings

2 pounds beets (about 6 medium-large), peeled and sliced ¼-inch thick

1½ cups orange juice

¼ teaspoon salt

⅛ teaspoon ground white pepper

¼ teaspoon ground cinnamon

¼ teaspoon ground ginger

⅛ teaspoon ground cloves

¼ cup white wine vinegar

2 medium sweet onions, thinly sliced

1. Place the beets, orange juice, salt, and spices in a 2-quart pot, and bring to a boil over high heat. Reduce the heat to medium-low, cover, and simmer for 25 minutes, or until the beets are tender.

2. Remove the pot from the heat, and let the beets cool slightly. Add the vinegar and onions, and toss to mix well.

3. Transfer the mixture to a shallow dish, cover, and chill for 8 hours or overnight before serving.

NUTRITIONAL FACTS (PER ⅔-CUP SERVING)

Calories: 58	Fat: 0.2 g	Protein: 1.8 g
Cholesterol: 0 mg	Fiber: 1.8 g	Sodium: 134 mg

Broccoli and Basil Pasta Salad

1. Cook the pasta until barely al dente according to package directions. Add the broccoli and carrots to the pot, and cook for another 30 to 60 seconds, or just until the broccoli turns bright green and is crisp-tender. Drain the pasta and vegetables, rinse with cold water, and drain again. Transfer the mixture to a large bowl, and toss in the red pepper.

2. In a small bowl, combine the dressing ingredients, and stir to mix. Pour the dressing over the pasta and vegetables, and toss gently to mix well.

3. Cover the salad and chill for at least 2 hours or overnight before serving.

Yield: 10 servings

8 ounces rotini or penne pasta

2½ cups fresh broccoli florets

⅔ cup diagonally sliced carrots (about 1 large)

½ cup matchstick-sized pieces red bell pepper (about ½ medium)

DRESSING

½ cup nonfat or reduced-fat mayonnaise

⅓ cup nonfat sour cream

¼ cup orange juice

1 tablespoon mustard

1 tablespoon finely chopped fresh basil, or 1 teaspoon dried

¼ teaspoon ground white pepper

NUTRITIONAL FACTS (PER ¾-CUP SERVING)		
Calories: 115	Fat: 0.5 g	Protein: 4 g
Cholesterol: 0 mg	Fiber: 1.5 g	Sodium: 140 mg

California Carrot Salad

1. Place the carrots and raisins in a large bowl, and toss to mix well.

2. Combine the dressing ingredients in small bowl, and stir to mix. Pour the dressing over the carrot mixture, and toss to mix well.

3. Cover the salad and chill for several hours or overnight before serving.

Yield: 10 servings

6 cups grated carrots (about 12 medium)

1 cup golden raisins

DRESSING

⅓ cup frozen orange juice concentrate, thawed

⅓ cup nonfat or reduced-fat mayonnaise

⅓ cup nonfat sour cream

NUTRITIONAL FACTS (PER ⅔-CUP SERVING)		
Calories: 105	Fat: 0.2 g	Protein: 1.4 g
Cholesterol: 0 mg	Fiber: 2.4 g	Sodium: 101 mg

Seven-Layer Slaw

Yield: 12 servings

2 teaspoons lemon juice

2 teaspoons sugar

1½ cups chopped peeled apples
   (about 1½ medium)

1 cup nonfat sour cream

1 cup reduced-fat or nonfat
   mayonnaise

6 cups shredded cabbage (about ½
   medium head)

1 can (8 ounces) sliced water
   chestnuts, drained

1 cup (about 6 ounces) frozen green
   peas, thawed

¾ cup shredded nonfat or
   reduced-fat Cheddar cheese

¼ cup chopped pecans (optional)

1. Combine the lemon juice and sugar in a small bowl. Add the apples, and toss to mix. Set aside.

2. Combine the sour cream and mayonnaise in a small bowl, and stir to mix well. Set aside.

3. To assemble the salad, place the cabbage in a 2½-quart glass serving bowl. Arrange the apple mixture in a layer over the cabbage, followed by a layer of water chestnuts and a layer of peas. Spread the sour cream mixture over the peas, and sprinkle the cheese over the sour cream. If desired, top with a sprinkling of nuts.

4. Cover the salad and chill for several hours or overnight. To serve, dip a serving spoon down through all of the layers so that each serving includes some of each ingredient.

NUTRITIONAL FACTS (PER ⅔-CUP SERVING)		
Calories: 81	Fat: 0.2 g	Protein: 4.2 g
Cholesterol: 2 mg	Fiber: 2 g	Sodium: 264 mg

Chinese Cucumber Salad

Yield: 8 servings

3 cups peeled, sliced cucumbers
   (about 3 medium)

1 medium onion, thinly sliced

DRESSING

¼ cup seasoned rice wine vinegar

1 tablespoon reduced-sodium soy
   sauce

1 teaspoon sesame oil

⅛ teaspoon ground white pepper

1. Place the cucumbers and onions in a shallow dish, and toss to mix.

2. Combine the dressing ingredients in a small bowl, and stir to mix. Pour the dressing over the vegetables, and stir to mix well.

3. Cover the salad and chill for several hours or overnight before serving.

NUTRITIONAL FACTS (PER ½-CUP SERVING)		
Calories: 29	Fat: 0.7 g	Protein: 1.1 g
Cholesterol: 0 mg	Fiber: 1.1 g	Sodium: 174 mg

Crowning Touches

Scan the shelves of your local grocery store, and you'll find a dazzling array of reduced-fat and nonfat salad dressings. Unfortunately, many commercial brands contain far too much sodium—sometimes more than 200 milligrams per tablespoon. Make your own dressing, though, and the result will not only be low in sodium and fat, but also full of the fresh-made flavor that only homemade dressings have.

Do croutons have a place on a low-fat salad? Certainly, many commercial brands don't. But if you use the recipe on page 78, you will be able to enjoy crunchy garlicky croutons without paying a high-fat price.

Sour Cream-Blue Cheese Dressing

1. Combine all of the ingredients except for ¼ cup of the blue cheese in a food processor or blender, and process for about 1 minute, or until the mixture is smooth. Stir in the remaining blue cheese.

2. Transfer the dressing to a covered container, and refrigerate for several hours before serving.

Yield: 1½ cups

½ cup nonfat sour cream

½ cup nonfat or reduced-fat mayonnaise

¼ cup white wine vinegar

2 cloves garlic

¼ teaspoon ground white pepper

½ cup crumbled blue cheese, divided

NUTRITIONAL FACTS (PER TABLESPOON)

Calories: 17	Fat: 0.6 g	Protein: 0.7 g
Cholesterol: 2 mg	Fiber: 0 g	Sodium: 96 mg

Honey Mustard Dressing

1. Combine all of the ingredients in a small bowl, and stir to mix well.

2. Transfer the dressing to a covered container, and refrigerate for several hours before serving.

Yield: 1⅛ cups

½ cup nonfat or reduced-fat mayonnaise

¼ cup honey

¼ cup mustard

2 tablespoons lemon juice

NUTRITIONAL FACTS (PER TABLESPOON)

Calories: 21	Fat: 0.2 g	Protein: 0.2 g
Cholesterol: 0 mg	Fiber: 0.1 g	Sodium: 119 mg

Creamy Italian Dressing

Yield: 2¹⁄₈ cups

¾ cup nonfat or reduced-fat
   mayonnaise

¾ cup skim milk

¼ cup red or white wine vinegar

3 cloves garlic

¼ teaspoon dried Italian seasoning

¼ teaspoon ground white pepper

½ cup grated nonfat or
   reduced-fat Parmesan cheese

1. Combine all of the ingredients in a food processor or blender, and process for about 1 minute, or until the mixture is smooth.

2. Transfer the dressing to a covered container, and refrigerate for several hours before serving.

NUTRITIONAL FACTS (PER TABLESPOON)

Calories: 10	Fat: 0 g	Protein: 0.7 g
Cholesterol: 1 mg	Fiber: 0 g	Sodium: 72 mg

Garlic and Herb Croutons

Yield: 4¹⁄₂ cups

2 tablespoons chicken or vegetable
   broth

2 tablespoons grated nonfat or
   reduced-fat Parmesan cheese

2 teaspoons crushed fresh garlic

¾ teaspoon dried Italian seasoning

6 cups French bread cubes

1. Combine the broth, cheese, garlic, and Italian seasoning in a small dish, and stir to mix well. Rub the mixture over the inside of a large bowl. Place the bread cubes in the bowl, and toss gently to coat the cubes with the garlic mixture.

2. Coat a large baking sheet with nonstick cooking spray. Arrange the bread cubes in a single layer on the sheet, and bake at 350°F for 16 to 18 minutes, or until the croutons are lightly browned and crisp.

3. Turn the oven off, and let the croutons cool in the oven with the door ajar for 30 minutes. Store in an airtight container until ready to use.

NUTRITIONAL FACTS (PER 3-TABLESPOON SERVING)

Calories: 21	Fat: 0.2 g	Protein: 0.8 g
Cholesterol: 0 mg	Fiber: 0.2 g	Sodium: 51 mg

Fresh Tomato Dressing

1. Combine all of the ingredients in a food processor or blender, and process for about 1 minute, or until the mixture is smooth.

2. Transfer the dressing to a covered container, and refrigerate for several hours before serving.

Yield: 1½ cups

1½ medium ripe tomatoes, chopped

¼ cup chopped onion

¼ cup plus 2 tablespoons red wine vinegar

2 tablespoons honey

1 tablespoon olive oil (optional)

1 tablespoon chopped fresh parsley, or 1 teaspoon dried

3 cloves garlic

2 teaspoons ground paprika

¾ teaspoon salt

¼ teaspoon ground black pepper

NUTRITIONAL FACTS (PER TABLESPOON)

Calories: 8	Fat: 0 g	Protein: 0.1 g
Cholesterol: 0 mg	Fiber: 0.1 g	Sodium: 68 mg

South of the Border Salad

1. Place the beans, corn, bell pepper, and onion in a large bowl, and toss to mix well.

2. Combine the dressing ingredients in small bowl, and stir to mix. Pour the dressing over the bean mixture, and toss to mix well.

3. Cover the salad and chill for several hours or overnight before serving.

Yield: 6 servings

1 can (1 pound) black beans, rinsed and drained

2 cups (about 12 ounces) frozen whole kernel corn, thawed

½ cup chopped green bell pepper

¼ cup chopped onion

DRESSING

½ cup picante sauce

1–2 tablespoons minced fresh cilantro

1 teaspoon crushed fresh garlic

½ teaspoon ground cumin

1 teaspoon sugar

NUTRITIONAL FACTS (PER ⅔-CUP SERVING)

Calories: 123	Fat: 0.9 g	Protein: 6.3 g
Cholesterol: 0 mg	Fiber: 6.1 g	Sodium: 222 mg

Dillicious Potato Salad

Yield: 9 servings

2 pounds unpeeled potatoes (about 6
  medium)

1 cup (about 6 ounces) frozen green
  peas, thawed

⅓ cup finely chopped carrot

⅓ cup chopped onion

DRESSING

¼ cup plus 2 tablespoons nonfat sour
  cream

¼ cup plus 2 tablespoons nonfat or
  reduced-fat mayonnaise

1 tablespoon lemon juice

1 tablespoon Dijon mustard

¼ teaspoon ground white pepper

1 tablespoon finely chopped fresh dill,
  or 1 teaspoon dried

1. Cut the potatoes in ¾-inch pieces, and place in a microwave or stove-top steamer. Cover and cook at high power or over medium-high heat for 8 to 10 minutes, or until tender. Rinse with cool water and drain.

2. Place the potatoes in a large bowl. Add the peas, carrots, and onions, and toss gently to mix.

3. Combine the dressing ingredients in a small bowl, and stir to mix well. Pour the dressing over the potato mixture, and toss gently to mix.

4. Cover the salad and chill for at least 2 hours or overnight before serving.

NUTRITIONAL FACTS (PER ¾-CUP SERVING)

Calories: 145	Fat: 0.2 g	Protein: 3.7 g
Cholesterol: 0 mg	Fiber: 3.4 g	Sodium: 146 mg

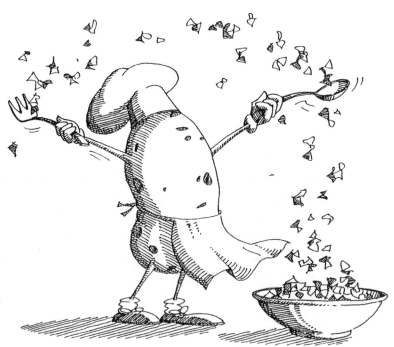

Italian Pasta Salad

This is a basic salad that can be varied in many ways.

Yield: 8 servings

1. Cook the pasta al dente according to package directions. Drain, rinse with cold water, and drain again.

2. Place the pasta in a large bowl. Add the tomato, scallions, and olives, and toss to mix well. Add the Italian dressing and cheese, and toss to mix well.

3. Cover the salad and chill for at least 2 hours or overnight before serving.

8 ounces rotini or penne pasta

1 medium tomato, chopped

$\frac{1}{4}$ cup sliced scallions

$\frac{1}{4}$ cup sliced black olives

$\frac{1}{3}$ cup bottled nonfat Italian dressing

$\frac{1}{4}$ cup grated nonfat or reduced-fat Parmesan cheese

---

NUTRITIONAL FACTS (PER $\frac{3}{4}$-CUP SERVING)

Calories: 130	Fat: 0.9 g	Protein: 4.9 g
Cholesterol: 2 mg	Fiber: 1.1 g	Sodium: 226 mg

Variations

For variety, add any of the following:

- $\frac{1}{2}$ cup chopped seeded cucumber and $\frac{1}{2}$ cup chopped red bell pepper
- 1 cup lightly steamed broccoli florets
- $\frac{3}{4}$ pound cooked shrimp
- 1 cup chopped artichoke hearts
- $\frac{1}{2}$ cup zucchini cut into matchstick-sized pieces and $\frac{1}{2}$ cup grated carrot
- 1 cup cooked or canned kidney, garbanzo, or white beans

Great Garbanzo Salad

Yield: 8 servings

1⅓ cups water

⅔ cup uncooked couscous

1 can (15 ounces) garbanzo beans, rinsed and drained

1 medium tomato, diced

1 medium cucumber, peeled, seeded, and diced

⅓ cup chopped purple onion

2 tablespoons minced fresh parsley

DRESSING

¼ cup red or white wine vinegar

1 tablespoon olive oil (optional)

1 teaspoon dried oregano

⅛ teaspoon ground black pepper

1. To cook the couscous, place the water in a 1-quart pot, and bring to a boil over high heat. Stir in the couscous, cover, and remove the pot from the heat. Let sit for 5 minutes, or until the water is absorbed. Uncover the pot, and set aside to cool.

2. Place the couscous, garbanzo beans, tomato, cucumber, onion, and parsley in a large bowl, and toss to mix well.

3. Combine the dressing ingredients in a small bowl, and stir to mix. Pour the dressing over the couscous mixture, and toss to mix well.

4. Cover the salad and chill for at least 2 hours or overnight before serving.

NUTRITIONAL FACTS (PER ⅔-CUP SERVING)		
Calories: 109	Fat: 0.9 g	Protein: 4.7 g
Cholesterol: 0 mg	Fiber: 2.5 g	Sodium: 90 mg

Rainbow Fruit Salad

Yield: 5 servings

1 cup sliced fresh strawberries

1 cup cubed cantaloupe

1 cup diced kiwi fruit

1 cup sliced bananas

1 cup fresh blueberries

DRESSING

2 tablespoons frozen orange juice concentrate, thawed

1 tablespoon honey

¾ teaspoon poppy seeds

1. Place the fruit in a large bowl, and toss to mix.

2. Combine the dressing ingredients in a small bowl, and stir to mix. Pour the dressing over the fruit, and toss to mix well.

3. Cover the salad and chill for 1 to 3 hours before serving.

NUTRITIONAL FACTS (PER 1-CUP SERVING)		
Calories: 121	Fat: 0.8 g	Protein: 1.7 g
Cholesterol: 0 mg	Fiber: 4 g	Sodium: 7 mg

Rosemary Rice Salad

1. Place the rice, broccoli, carrots, celery, and raisins in a large bowl, and toss to mix well.

2. Combine the dressing ingredients in a small bowl, and stir to mix. Pour the dressing over the rice mixture, and toss to mix well.

3. Cover the salad and chill for at least 2 hours or overnight before serving.

Yield: 8 servings

3 cups cooked brown rice

1 cup finely chopped fresh broccoli stems

½ cup grated carrots

⅓ cup finely chopped celery

¼ cup dark or golden raisins

DRESSING

¼ cup orange juice

2 tablespoons white wine vinegar

1 tablespoon olive oil (optional)

1 teaspoon crushed fresh garlic

1 tablespoon chopped fresh rosemary, or 1 teaspoon dried

½ teaspoon ground ginger

¼ teaspoon salt

NUTRITIONAL FACTS (PER ⅔-CUP SERVING)

Calories: 107	Fat: 0.7 g	Protein: 2.5 g
Cholesterol: 0 mg	Fiber: 2.1 g	Sodium: 81 mg

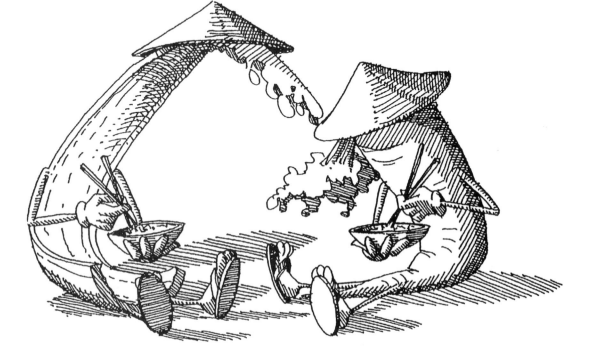

Curried Rice and Bean Salad

Yield: 8 servings

3 cups cooked brown rice

1 can (1 pound) red kidney beans, rinsed and drained

½ cup chopped green bell pepper

½ cup thinly sliced celery

⅓ cup thinly sliced scallions

¼ cup dark raisins

DRESSING

⅓ cup nonfat or reduced-fat mayonnaise

⅓ cup plain nonfat yogurt

1–2 teaspoons curry powder

⅛ teaspoon ground black pepper

1. Place the rice, beans, bell pepper, celery, scallions, and raisins in a large bowl, and toss to mix well.

2. Combine the dressing ingredients in a small bowl, and stir to mix. Pour the dressing over the rice mixture, and toss to mix well.

3. Cover the salad and chill for at least 2 hours or overnight before serving.

NUTRITIONAL FACTS (PER ¾-CUP SERVING)

Calories: 163	Fat: 0.9 g	Protein: 6.2 g
Cholesterol: 0 mg	Fiber: 4.9 g	Sodium: 209 mg

Winter Fruit Salad

Yield: 8 servings

3 cups diced unpeeled red delicious apples

1½ cups sliced celery

1 cup seedless green grapes, halved

½ cup dark raisins

DRESSING

¼ cup nonfat mayonnaise

¼ cup nonfat sour cream

1. Combine the apples, celery, grapes, and raisins in a large bowl, and toss to mix well.

2. Combine the dressing ingredients in a small bowl, and stir to mix. Pour the dressing over the apple mixture, and toss to mix well.

3. Cover the salad and chill for 1 to 3 hours before serving.

NUTRITIONAL FACTS (PER ¾-CUP SERVING)

Calories: 82	Fat: 0.3 g	Protein: 0.9 g
Cholesterol: 0 mg	Fiber: 1.6 g	Sodium: 94 mg

7. Smart Vegetable Side Dishes

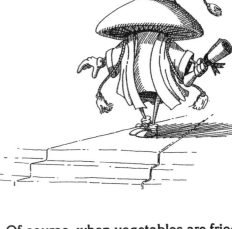

Mom was right when she told you to eat your vegetables. The most nutrient-rich of all foods, veggies are loaded with vitamins, minerals, and fiber—all powerful preventive medicines in the fight against cancer, heart disease, and many other disorders. As for fat and cholesterol, vegetables contain neither. And they're low in calories, too. A half cup of nonstarchy vegetables like asparagus, broccoli, cauliflower, green beans, or summer squash has a mere 25 calories. Even starchy vegetables like potatoes, corn, and peas have only about 80 calories per half cup. Compare this with the other foods on your plate—a three-ounce portion of roast chicken can have anywhere from 140 to 250 calories, for instance—and it's clear that veggies are a calorie counter's best friend.

Because of the many health benefits of vegetables, it is currently recommended that a healthy diet contain at least three to five servings of veggies a day. This isn't as much as it may seem, as a serving is only one half cup of cooked vegetables, or one cup of raw leafy vegetables. In other words, two good-sized portions of your favorite vegetables at dinner time will probably fulfill your minimum daily requirement.

Of course, when vegetables are fried in oil or swimming in butter or fat-laden sauces, nutritionally, they are not much better than a bowl of chips. But once you know the secrets of fat-free cooking, you will find that there are many ways to make vegetables tasty and appealing without butter, margarine, or other high-fat foods.

The recipes in this chapter use herbs, spices, and a variety of other ingredients to give vegetables flavor without fat—and without an unhealthy dose of sodium, too. Thanks to products like nonfat cheese and nonfat sour cream, you will find that even home-style vegetable casseroles and creamy Cheddar cheese toppings can be prepared with little or no fat. As an added bonus, these recipes often replace boiling with steaming, stir-frying, and other cooking techniques that minimize nutrient loss while keeping veggies bright in color and bursting with garden-fresh flavor. The result? Your vegetable dishes will be not just tasty, but also rich in the vitamins, minerals, and fiber that make them such an important part of your daily diet. Mom would be proud!

Down-Home Lima Beans

Yield: 9 servings

2 cups dried large lima beans, cleaned and soaked (page 148)

5 cups unsalted chicken broth or water

1 medium onion, chopped

1½ teaspoons ham or chicken bouillon granules

1 bay leaf

2 teaspoons dried sage

¼ teaspoon ground black pepper

1. Combine all of the ingredients in a 2½-quart pot, and bring to a boil over high heat. Reduce the heat to low, cover, and simmer, stirring occasionally, for 1 hour and 30 minutes, or until the beans are soft and the liquid is thick. Periodically check the pot during cooking, and add a little more broth or water if needed.

2. Remove the pot from the heat, and discard the bay leaf. Serve hot.

NUTRITIONAL FACTS (PER ⅔-CUP SERVING)

Calories: 140	Fat: 0.2 g	Protein: 8.5 g
Cholesterol: 0 mg	Fiber: 8 g	Sodium: 175 mg

Country-Style Green Beans

Yield: 6 servings

1½ pounds fresh green beans, cut into 1-inch pieces

½ cup water

1¼ teaspoons ham bouillon granules, or 3 ounces ham (at least 97% lean), diced

1 teaspoon dry mustard

⅛ teaspoon ground black pepper

1. Combine the green beans, water, bouillon granules or ham, mustard, and pepper in a 2½-quart pot, and bring to a boil over medium heat. Reduce the heat to low, and simmer uncovered, stirring occasionally, for 2 to 3 minutes, or until the beans turn bright green.

2. Cover the pot, and simmer, stirring occasionally, for 15 to 20 minutes, or until the beans are tender. Serve immediately.

NUTRITIONAL FACTS (PER ⅔-CUP SERVING)

Calories: 37	Fat: 0.2 g	Protein: 2.2 g
Cholesterol: 0 mg	Fiber: 3.9 g	Sodium: 176 mg

Mom's Broccoli Casserole

1. To make the sauce, combine $\frac{1}{4}$ cup of the milk and all of the milk powder and cornstarch in a small dish. Stir to mix well, and set aside.

2. Place the water or broth, mushrooms, onions, thyme, and pepper in a 2½-quart saucepan, and place the pan over medium heat. Cook and stir for about 2 minutes, or until the vegetables are tender and most of the liquid has evaporated.

3. Add the remaining 1¼ cups of milk to the pot, and continue to cook and stir just until the mixture starts to boil. Stir the cornstarch mixture once, and add it to the pot. Cook and stir for a minute or 2, or until the sauce is thickened and bubbly.

4. Remove the pot from the heat, and stir the broccoli, rice, and cheese into the sauce. Coat a 2-quart casserole dish with nonstick cooking spray, and spread the mixture evenly in the dish. Sprinkle the crumbs over the top of the mixture, and spray the crumbs lightly with nonstick cooking spray.

5. Bake at 350°F for 50 minutes to 1 hour, or until the top is golden brown and the edges are bubbly. Remove the dish from the oven, and let sit for 5 minutes before serving.

Yield: 8 servings

2 packages (10 ounces each) frozen chopped broccoli, thawed and squeezed dry

1½ cups cooked brown rice

1½ cups shredded nonfat or reduced-fat Cheddar cheese

2 tablespoons finely ground fat-free cracker crumbs

Nonstick cooking spray

SAUCE

1½ cups skim milk, divided

¼ cup instant nonfat dry milk powder

1 tablespoon plus 1½ teaspoons cornstarch

1 tablespoon water or unsalted chicken broth

½ cup finely chopped fresh mushrooms

½ cup finely chopped onion

¼ teaspoon dried thyme

¼ teaspoon ground black pepper

NUTRITIONAL FACTS (PER ¾-CUP SERVING)

Calories: 133	Fat: 0.5 g	Protein: 12.7 g
Cholesterol: 5 mg	Fiber: 3 g	Sodium: 248 mg

FAT-FREE COOKING TIP

Sautéing Without Fat

When sautéing vegetables, replace part or all of the fat usually used with broth, sherry, white wine, or another liquid. For every tablespoon of butter you eliminate, you will save 100 calories and 11 grams of fat. Each time you eliminate a tablespoon of oil, you will save 120 calories and 14 grams of fat.

Cauliflower au Gratin

Yield: 5 servings

1 package (1 pound) frozen
  cauliflower florets, thawed and
  drained

1 recipe Cheddar Cheese Sauce (page
  96)

2 tablespoons finely ground fat-free
  cracker crumbs (onion or herb
  flavor)

Nonstick cooking spray

1. Combine the cauliflower and cheese sauce in a large bowl, and toss to mix well. Coat a 1½-quart casserole dish with nonstick cooking spray, and spread the mixture evenly in the dish. Sprinkle the crumbs over the top of the mixture, and spray the crumbs lightly with nonstick cooking spray.

2. Bake at 350°F for 30 minutes, or until the top is browned and the edges are bubbly. Remove the dish from the oven, and let sit for 5 minutes before serving.

NUTRITIONAL FACTS (PER ¾-CUP SERVING)

Calories: 80	Fat: 0.3 g	Protein: 9 g
Cholesterol: 4 mg	Fiber: 1.8 g	Sodium: 221 mg

Carrot-Rice Casserole

Yield: 8 servings

3 cups grated carrots (about 6
  medium)

3 cups cooked brown rice

½ cup finely chopped onion

1 tablespoon minced fresh parsley, or
   1 teaspoon dried

1 tablespoon minced fresh savory, or
   1 teaspoon dried

¼ teaspoon salt

1½ cups evaporated skim milk

½ cup fat-free egg substitute

3 tablespoons grated nonfat or
   reduced-fat Parmesan cheese

1. Combine the carrots, rice, onions, herbs, and salt in a large bowl, and stir to mix well. Add the milk and egg substitute, and stir to mix. Coat a 2-quart casserole dish with nonstick cooking spray, and spread the mixture evenly in the dish. Sprinkle the cheese over the top.

2. Bake at 350°F for 50 minutes to 1 hour, or until a sharp knife inserted in the center of the dish comes out clean. Remove the dish from the oven, and let sit for 5 minutes before serving.

NUTRITIONAL FACTS (PER ¾-CUP SERVING)

Calories: 154	Fat: 0.8 g	Protein: 8.5 g
Cholesterol: 3 mg	Fiber: 2.6 g	Sodium: 184 mg

Top: Pasta Fagioli Soup (page 64)
Center: Spanish Bean Soup (page 72)
Bottom: Tomato Florentine Soup (page 71)

Top Right: Great Garbanzo Salad (page 82)
Center Left: Italian Pasta Salad (page 81)
Center Right: Broccoli and Basil Pasta Salad (page 75)
Bottom Left: Antipasto Salad (page 74)

Top: **Stuffed Eggplant Extraordinaire (page 91)**
Center: **Mom's Broccoli Casserole (page 87)**
Bottom: **Cranapple Acorn Squash (page 95)**

Top: Pasta With Crab and Asparagus (page 105)
Center: Bow Ties With Spicy Artichoke Sauce (page 106)
Bottom: Pasta Primavera (page 107)

Top: Lasagna Roll-Ups (page 109)
Bottom Left: Florentine Stuffed Shells (page 110)
Bottom Right: Light and Lazy Lasagna (page 108)

Top Left: Shepherd's Pie (page 131)
Top Right: Crispy Cajun Chicken (page 116)
Bottom: Lemon-Herb Chicken With Vegetables (page 112)

Top: Chicken Enchiladas (page 118)
Center: Old-Fashioned Beef Stew (page 126)
Bottom: Foil-Baked Flounder (page 122)

Top: Saucy Stuffed Peppers (page 129)
Center: Mama Mia Meat Loaf (page 127)
Bottom: Breast of Turkey Provençal (page 120)

Cabbage and Potato Curry

Yield: 6 servings

1. Combine the potatoes and broth in a large nonstick skillet. Place the skillet over medium-low heat, cover, and cook, stirring occasionally, for about 10 minutes, or until the potatoes are tender.

2. Add the cabbage and curry to the skillet, and stir to mix. Cover and cook, stirring occasionally, for 7 to 9 minutes, or until the cabbage is tender. Serve hot.

2 medium unpeeled potatoes, sliced $\frac{1}{4}$ inch thick

$\frac{1}{2}$ cup chicken or vegetable broth

$\frac{1}{2}$ medium head cabbage, halved and cut into 1-inch pieces

2–3 teaspoons curry powder

NUTRITIONAL FACTS (PER $\frac{3}{4}$-CUP SERVING)

Calories: 84	Fat: 0.3 g	Protein: 2.8 g
Cholesterol: 0 mg	Fiber: 2.9 g	Sodium: 83 mg

Cooking Country Style

Southern-style vegetables are typically seasoned with bacon, lard, or ham hocks. Delicious? Absolutely! Healthy? As you might expect, these dishes are loaded with fat and salt. Fortunately, a variety of ingredients can be substituted for the usual Southern flavorings, resulting in mouthwatering dishes that are untraditionally low in fat. Here are some ideas:

❒ *Bouillon granules.* Ham bouillon granules can be added to a pot of beans or cabbage as a fat-free alternative to ham or bacon. Look for a brand like Goya, which is usually located in the ethnic foods section of grocery stores. Chicken- and vegetable-flavored bouillons are still another option. What about sodium? A teaspoon of the granules typically contains 1,000 milligrams of sodium—about half the amount in a teaspoon of salt. You can eliminate salt worries, though, by choosing a brand like Vogue Vege Base, a vegetable bouillon made mostly of powdered vegetables. Do keep in mind that most bouillons contain monosodium glutamate (MSG), and read labels carefully if you want to avoid this ingredient.

❒ *Lean ham.* Many hams—both turkey and pork—are very low in fat. Look for brands that are at least 97 percent lean. Then dice the ham and add small amounts to bean soups, greens, and other vegetable dishes.

❒ *Smoked turkey sausage.* Like lean ham, this product will add a smoky flavor to a variety of dishes. Look for brands like Healthy Choice, which is 97 percent lean, and use the sausage as you would lean ham.

❒ *Smoked turkey parts.* This is a great alternative to ham hocks. Add chunks of skinless smoked turkey to bean soups, green beans, and other vegetables.

❒ *Herbs and spices.* Because sage, fennel, and thyme are traditionally used to flavor sausage, these spices can be used instead of meat to add a country-style taste to bean soups and many vegetable dishes.

❒ *Vinegar.* A splash of vinegar or lemon juice tossed into vegetables just before serving adds zip, reducing the need for salty seasonings. Experiment with different types of vinegar, such as cider, white wine, red wine, rice wine, malt, and balsamic.

Confetti Corn Pudding

Yield: 6 servings

Puréed corn, rather than cream, adds richness to this colorful dish.

1 pound frozen whole kernel corn, thawed, or 3⅓ cups fresh, divided

⅓ cup chopped onion

¾ cup plus 2 tablespoons skim milk

½ cup fat-free egg substitute

2 tablespoons unbleached flour

¼ teaspoon salt

⅛ teaspoon ground black pepper

1 tablespoon chopped fresh parsley, or 1 teaspoon dried

¼ cup finely chopped green bell pepper

¼ cup finely chopped red bell pepper

1. Place 1 cup of the corn and all of the onion, milk, egg substitute, flour, salt, and pepper in a blender or food processor. Process for 1 minute, or until the mixture is smooth. Add the parsley, and process for an additional 10 seconds.

2. Place the corn mixture in a large bowl, and add the remaining corn kernels and the peppers. Stir to mix well.

3. Coat a 1½-quart casserole dish with nonstick cooking spray, and pour the corn mixture into the dish. Bake at 350°F for 1 hour, or until a sharp knife inserted midway between the center of the dish and the rim comes out clean. Remove the dish from the oven, and let sit for 5 minutes before serving.

NUTRITIONAL FACTS (PER ⅔-CUP SERVING)		
Calories: 98	Fat: 0.2 g	Protein: 5.6 g
Cholesterol: 0 mg	Fiber: 2.1 g	Sodium: 141 mg

Skillet Squash and Onions

Yield: 6 servings

1½ pounds zucchini or yellow squash (about 4–5 medium zucchini or 8–10 medium squash)

1 medium yellow onion, sliced ¼-inch thick

2 tablespoons water

2 teaspoons butter-flavored sprinkles

¼ teaspoon ground black pepper

1 tablespoon minced fresh dill, or 1 teaspoon dried

1. Cut each squash in half lengthwise; then cut each half into ¼-inch-thick slices. (There should be about 6 cups of squash. Adjust the amount if necessary.)

2. Place the squash and onions in a large nonstick skillet. Sprinkle the water, butter-flavored sprinkles, pepper, and dill over the top, and place the skillet over medium heat. Cover and cook, stirring occasionally, for 7 to 9 minutes, or just until the vegetables are tender. Serve hot.

NUTRITIONAL FACTS (PER ⅔-CUP SERVING)		
Calories: 25	Fat: 0.2 g	Protein: 1.5 g
Cholesterol: 0 mg	Fiber: 1.6 g	Sodium: 30 mg

Stuffed Eggplant Extraordinaire

1. Tear the bread into pieces, and place the pieces in a blender or food processor. Process into fine crumbs, and set aside.

2. Cut each eggplant in half lengthwise, and scoop out and reserve the flesh, leaving a $^3/_8$-inch-thick shell. Trim a small piece off the bottom of each shell, if necessary, to allow each half to sit upright. Set aside.

3. Coat a large skillet with nonstick cooking spray. Finely chop the removed eggplant, and transfer to the skillet. Add the tomato, bell pepper, onion, celery, salt, and black pepper to the skillet, and place over medium heat. Cover and cook, stirring occasionally, for 5 minutes, or until the vegetables are almost tender.

4. Remove the skillet from the heat, and stir in the bread crumbs and parsley. Divide the eggplant mixture among the 4 hollowed-out eggplant shells.

5. Coat a shallow baking dish with nonstick cooking spray, and arrange the stuffed shells in the dish. Sprinkle $1^1/_2$ teaspoons of cheese over the top of each stuffed shell, and bake at 350°F for 25 minutes, or until the filling is heated through and the top is golden brown.

Yield: 4 servings

2 slices whole wheat bread

2 small eggplants (about 8 ounces each)

1 medium tomato, finely chopped

$^1/_3$ cup finely chopped green bell pepper

$^1/_3$ cup finely chopped onion

$^1/_3$ cup finely chopped celery

$^1/_8$ teaspoon salt

$^1/_4$ teaspoon ground black pepper

2 tablespoons minced fresh parsley, or 2 teaspoons dried

2 tablespoons grated nonfat or reduced-fat Parmesan cheese

NUTRITIONAL FACTS (PER SERVING)		
Calories: 75	Fat: 0.8 g	Protein: 4.4 g
Cholesterol: 1 mg	Fiber: 4.5 g	Sodium: 163 mg

Swiss Onion Bake

Yield: 8 servings

1½ pounds mild sweet onions (about 4 medium)

1 tablespoon minced fresh parsley, or 1 teaspoon dried

2 tablespoons dry sherry or unsalted chicken broth

1 cup evaporated skim milk

1 cup fat-free egg substitute

¼ teaspoon ground white pepper

1 cup shredded nonfat or reduced-fat Swiss cheese

4 slices uncooked turkey bacon, cut in half (optional)

1. Cut the onions into thin wedges. Coat a large skillet with nonstick cooking spray, and add the onions, parsley, and sherry or broth. Place over medium heat, and cook, stirring constantly, for about 5 minutes, or until the onions are tender. (Add a little more sherry or broth if the skillet becomes too dry.) Remove the skillet from the heat, and set aside for a few minutes to cool slightly.

2. Stir the milk into the onion mixture. Add the egg substitute, pepper, and cheese, and stir to mix.

3. Coat a 2-quart casserole dish with nonstick cooking spray, and spread the onion mixture evenly in the dish. Arrange the bacon slices over the top, if desired, and bake at 375°F for 45 minutes, or until a sharp knife inserted in the center of the dish comes out clean. Remove the dish from the oven, and let sit for 5 minutes before serving.

NUTRITIONAL FACTS (PER ⅔-CUP SERVING)

Calories: 93	Fat: 0.2 g	Protein: 11 g
Cholesterol: 4 mg	Fiber: 1.5 g	Sodium: 189 mg

Stir-Fried Spinach

Yield: 4 servings

1 pound fresh spinach

1 teaspoon crushed fresh garlic

⅛ teaspoon ground black pepper

2 teaspoons lemon juice

1. Thoroughly wash the spinach and remove all tough stems. Shake off any excess water, but do not dry completely. Set aside.

2. Coat a large skillet with nonstick cooking spray, and preheat over medium-high heat. Add the garlic, and stir-fry for 30 seconds. Add the spinach and pepper, and stir-fry for about 2 minutes, or just until the spinach is wilted and tender.

3. Remove the skillet from the heat, and toss in the lemon juice. Serve hot.

NUTRITIONAL FACTS (PER ½-CUP SERVING)

Calories: 25	Fat: 0.4 g	Protein: 3.2 g
Cholesterol: 0 mg	Fiber: 3.1 g	Sodium: 89 mg

Golden Mashed Potatoes

1. Peel the rutabaga, and dice into $\frac{1}{2}$-inch cubes. Place the rutabaga in 3-quart pot, add enough water to barely cover, and bring to a boil over high heat. Reduce the heat to low, cover, and simmer, stirring occasionally, for 20 minutes, or until the rutabaga is almost tender.

2. Peel the potatoes, and cut into 1-inch pieces. Add the potatoes to the cooking rutabaga, adding water if needed to barely cover the vegetables. Bring to a second boil. Reduce the heat to low, cover, and simmer for 20 minutes, or until the vegetables are very tender.

3. Remove the pot from the heat, and drain off and reserve the cooking liquid. Add the salt and pepper to the vegetables, and mash or beat until smooth. Stir in the sour cream or yogurt, adding a little of the reserved cooking liquid if the mixture is too stiff. Serve hot.

Yield: 8 servings

1 medium rutabaga (about 1$\frac{1}{2}$ pounds)

1$\frac{1}{2}$ pounds baking potatoes (about 5–6 medium)

$\frac{1}{4}$ teaspoon salt

$\frac{1}{8}$ teaspoon ground white pepper

$\frac{1}{3}$ cup nonfat sour cream or plain nonfat yogurt

NUTRITIONAL FACTS (PER $\frac{2}{3}$-CUP SERVING)

Calories: 96	Fat: 0.2 g	Protein: 2.5 g
Cholesterol: 0 mg	Fiber: 3 g	Sodium: 97 mg

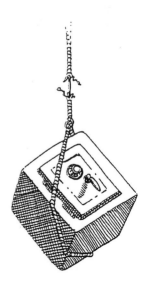

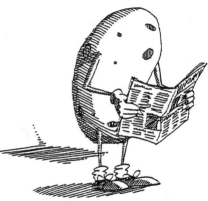

Hearty Oven Fries

Yield: 6 servings

1½ pounds unpeeled baking potatoes (about 3 extra large)

1 egg white, lightly beaten, or 2 tablespoons fat-free egg substitute

Nonstick cooking spray

COATING

2 teaspoons ground paprika

1 teaspoon garlic powder

¼ teaspoon salt

¼ teaspoon ground black pepper

1. Combine the coating ingredients in a small dish, and stir to mix well. Set aside.

2. Scrub the potatoes, dry well, and cut into ½-inch-thick strips. Place the potatoes in a large bowl. Pour the egg white or egg substitute over the potatoes, and toss to coat evenly. Sprinkle the coating over the potatoes, and toss again to coat.

3. Coat a large baking sheet with nonstick cooking spray, and arrange the potatoes in a single layer on the sheet, making sure that the potato strips are not touching one another. Spray the tops lightly with cooking spray, and bake at 400°F for 25 to 30 minutes, or until nicely browned and tender. Serve hot.

NUTRITIONAL FACTS (PER SERVING)		
Calories: 129	Fat: 0.3 g	Protein: 3.3 g
Cholesterol: 0 mg	Fiber: 2.7 g	Sodium: 98 mg

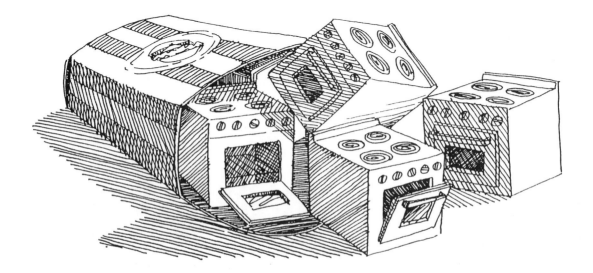

Stuffed Acorn Squash

Yield: 4 servings

1. Cut each squash in half crosswise, and scoop out and discard the seeds. Trim a small piece off the bottom of each squash half, if necessary, to allow the squash to sit upright.

2. Combine the remaining ingredients in a medium-sized bowl, and stir to mix well. Divide the mixture among the squash shells.

3. Coat a shallow baking dish with nonstick cooking spray, and arrange the stuffed shells in the dish. Cover the dish with aluminum foil, and bake at 350°F for 50 minutes to 1 hour, or until the squash are tender. Serve hot.

2 medium acorn squash (about 1 pound each)

1 cup cooked brown rice or bulgur wheat

1 medium tart apple, peeled and finely chopped

¼ cup thinly sliced celery

¼ cup finely chopped onion

¼ cup dark raisins

1 tablespoon butter-flavored sprinkles

¾ teaspoon dried thyme

NUTRITIONAL FACTS (PER SERVING)

Calories: 208	Fat: 0.8 g	Protein: 3.7 g
Cholesterol: 0 mg	Fiber: 9.5 g	Sodium: 77 mg

Cranapple Acorn Squash

Yield: 4 servings

1. Cut each squash in half crosswise, and scoop out and discard the seeds. Trim a small piece off the bottom of each squash half, if necessary, to allow the squash to sit upright.

2. Combine the apples, cranberries, raisins, brown sugar, and pecans, if desired, in a medium-sized bowl, and stir to mix well. Divide the mixture among the squash shells, and sprinkle a pinch of nutmeg over each stuffed shell.

3. Coat a shallow baking dish with nonstick cooking spray, and arrange the stuffed shells in the dish. Cover the dish with aluminum foil, and bake at 350°F for 50 minutes to 1 hour, or until the squash are tender. Serve hot.

2 medium acorn squash (about 1 pound each)

2 cups finely chopped peeled apple (about 3 medium)

½ cup coarsely chopped fresh or frozen (do not thaw) cranberries

¼ cup golden raisins

3 tablespoons light brown sugar

2 tablespoons chopped pecans (optional)

¼ teaspoon ground nutmeg

NUTRITIONAL FACTS (PER SERVING)

Calories: 183	Fat: 0.4 g	Protein: 2.3 g
Cholesterol: 0 mg	Fiber: 8.8 g	Sodium: 7 mg

Sauce It Up!

Vegetables blanketed with buttery or cheesy sauces are *not* what the doctor ordered. But take heart. Made properly, creamy rich-tasting sauces can still adorn your favorite veggies. Here are some ideas for fabulous fat-free toppings.

Cheddar Cheese Sauce

Yield: 1¼ cups

2 tablespoons unbleached flour

1 cup skim milk, divided

⅛ teaspoon ground white pepper

¾ cup shredded nonfat processed Cheddar cheese, or ¾ cup shredded reduced-fat Cheddar cheese

1. Combine the flour, ¼ cup of the milk, and the pepper in a small jar with a tight-fitting lid. Shake to mix well, and set aside.

2. Place the remaining ¾ cup of milk in a 1-quart saucepan. Place over medium heat, and cook, stirring constantly, until the mixture starts to boil. Stir in the flour mixture, and continue to cook and stir for a few seconds, or until the sauce is thickened and bubbly.

3. Reduce the heat to low, add the cheese, and continue to stir until the cheese melts. Serve hot over steamed broccoli, cauliflower, asparagus, potatoes, or other vegetables.

NUTRITIONAL FACTS (PER TABLESPOON)

Calories: 13	Fat: 0 g	Protein: 1.9 g
Cholesterol: 1 mg	Fiber: 0 g	Sodium: 51 mg

Honey Mustard Sauce

Yield: 1¼ cups

½ cup nonfat or reduced-fat mayonnaise

¼ cup honey

¼ cup mustard

¼ cup lemon juice

1. Combine all of the ingredients in a 1-quart saucepan, and stir to mix well. Place over medium-low heat, and cook, stirring constantly, just until the sauce is heated through.

2. Serve hot over steamed broccoli, cauliflower, asparagus, or other vegetables.

NUTRITIONAL FACTS (PER TABLESPOON)

Calories: 20	Fat: 0.1 g	Protein: 0.2 g
Cholesterol: 0 mg	Fiber: 0.1 g	Sodium: 107 mg

Creamy Lemon Sauce

This sauce can beautifully replace hollandaise in any of your favorite recipes.

Yield: 1½ cups

1 cup skim milk

¼ cup instant nonfat dry milk powder

1 tablespoon plus 1½ teaspoons cornstarch

½ teaspoon salt

⅛ teaspoon ground white pepper

1 pinch ground nutmeg

¼ cup fat-free egg substitute

3 tablespoons lemon juice

2 teaspoons freshly grated lemon rind

1. Place the milk, milk powder, cornstarch, salt, pepper, and nutmeg in a 1-quart saucepan, and stir until the cornstarch and milk powder are dissolved. Place over medium-low heat, and cook, stirring constantly, until the sauce is thickened and bubbly. Reduce the heat to low.

2. Place the egg substitute in a small bowl, and stir in ¼ cup of the hot milk mixture. Return the mixture to the pan, and continue to cook and stir for another minute, or until the mixture thickens slightly. Do not let the mixture boil.

3. Remove the pan from the heat, and slowly stir in the lemon juice and rind. Serve hot over steamed asparagus, broccoli, or cauliflower.

NUTRITIONAL FACTS (PER TABLESPOON)

Calories: 10 Fat: 0 g Protein: 0.9 g
Cholesterol: 0 mg Fiber: 0 g Sodium: 58 mg

Island Sweet Potatoes

Yield: 8 servings

2 cans (1 pound each) sweet potatoes, drained

1 can (8 ounces) crushed pineapple in juice, undrained

1 large firm but ripe banana, sliced

⅓ cup golden raisins or chopped dates

¼ teaspoon ground nutmeg

1¾ cups miniature marshmallows

1. Cut the sweet potatoes into bite-sized pieces, and place in a large bowl. Add the pineapple, including the juice, and the banana slices, raisins or dates, and nutmeg. Toss gently to mix.

2. Coat a 2-quart casserole dish with nonstick cooking spray, and spread the mixture evenly in the dish. Arrange the marshmallows over the top, and bake at 350°F for 35 to 40 minutes, or until the edges are bubbly and the topping is golden brown. Serve hot.

NUTRITIONAL FACTS (PER ⅔-CUP SERVING)

Calories: 156 Fat: 0.3 g Protein: 2.3 g
Cholesterol: 0 mg Fiber: 2 g Sodium: 68 mg

Baked Butternut Pudding

Yield: 8 servings

3 pounds butternut squash (about 2 medium)

2 cups apple juice

2 tablespoons light brown sugar

1 tablespoon plus 1 teaspoon butter-flavored sprinkles

1/2 teaspoon ground cinnamon

1/4 teaspoon ground nutmeg

1/2 cup fat-free egg substitute

TOPPING

3 tablespoons light brown sugar

3 tablespoons toasted wheat germ or finely chopped pecans

1. Peel and seed the squash, and cut the remaining flesh into cubes. Place the squash and the apple juice in a 4-quart pot, and bring to a boil over high heat. Reduce the heat to low, cover, and simmer, stirring occasionally, for 25 minutes, or until the squash is very tender.

2. Remove the pot from the heat, and drain off and discard the juice. Add the brown sugar, butter-flavored sprinkles, cinnamon, and nutmeg to the squash, and mash the mixture with a potato masher until smooth.

3. Place the egg substitute in a small bowl, and stir in 1/2 cup of the hot mashed squash. Return the mixture to the pot.

4. To make the topping, combine the topping ingredients in a small bowl, and stir to mix well. Set aside.

5. Coat a 2-quart casserole dish with nonstick cooking spray, and spread the squash mixture evenly in the dish. Sprinkle the topping over the squash, and bake at 350°F for 45 to 50 minutes, or until a sharp knife inserted in the center of the dish comes out clean. Remove the dish from the oven, and let sit for 5 minutes before serving.

NUTRITIONAL FACTS (PER 2/3-CUP SERVING)

Calories: 115	Fat: 0.6 g	Protein: 3.8 g
Cholesterol: 0 mg	Fiber: 4.5 g	Sodium: 43 mg

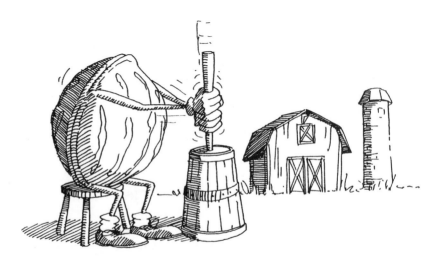

8. Pasta Mania

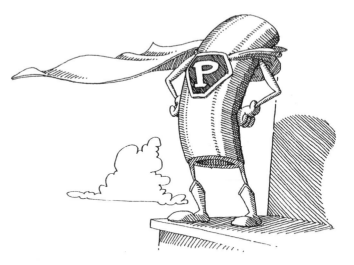

Need a low-fat meal in a matter of minutes? Think pasta. Contrary to popular belief, pasta is not fattening. One cup of cooked pasta—about two ounces dry—has only about two hundred calories and one gram of fat. Pasta is also loaded with energizing complex carbohydrates, and is so-dium-free. For the most nutrients, select whole grain pastas. Like whole grain breads, these pastas provide far more B vitamins, minerals, and fiber than do products made from refined white flour. As a bonus, whole grains lend pastas a nutty flavor that enhances any dish.

Why is pasta so often thought of as being fattening? The problem is not with the pasta—it's with what so often goes on top. Cream-enriched sauces, pools of olive oil or butter, gobs of high-fat cheese, and greasy sausages are just a few of the toppings that can turn a lean plate of pasta into a fat budget-busting nightmare. But can these fatty in-gredients be eliminated without sacrificing flavor? Absolutely. This chapter will show you how.

None of the recipes in this chapter requires any added fat. Instead, these recipes combine pasta with nonfat cheeses, skim milk, ultra-lean meats, seafood, vegetables, herbs and spices, and other wholesome ingredients. The result? Pasta creations that are every bit as tempting as their full-fat counterparts. And you'll be delighted to find that pasta is a snap to prepare. In fact, most of the dishes in this chapter can be whipped up in less than thirty minutes, making pasta a boon to the busy cook.

When reading through the following recipes, keep in mind that this is just a sampling of the many pasta dishes that can be made low-fat and luscious. Chapter 6 shows you how to blend pasta with fresh veggies and low-fat dressings to make delightful chilled salads. And later in this chapter, you'll learn the secrets of ingredient substitution that will allow you to turn any pasta dish, no matter how rich, into a low-fat delight. So the next time you need a delicious dinner in a hurry—or you're just in the mood for a satisfying plate of comfort food— boil up some pasta, and enjoy the pleasures of fat-free cooking.

Fettuccine Almost Alfredo

Yield: 5 servings

12 ounces fettuccine pasta

¾ cup grated nonfat or reduced-fat
  Parmesan cheese

SAUCE

1 cup nonfat ricotta cheese

¾ cup skim milk

1 tablespoon butter-flavored sprinkles

⅛ teaspoon ground white pepper

1. Cook the pasta al dente according to package directions. Drain well, return the pasta to the pot, and cover to keep warm.

2. While the pasta is cooking, combine all of the sauce ingredients in a blender or food processor, and process until smooth. Pour the mixture into a 1-quart saucepan, place over low heat, and cook, stirring constantly, just until the mixture is heated through. Do not allow the sauce to boil.

3. Pour the sauce over the pasta, add the Parmesan, and toss gently to mix well. Serve immediately.

NUTRITIONAL FACTS (PER 1⅓-CUP SERVING)

Calories: 342	Fat: 1.1 g	Protein: 22 g
Cholesterol: 20 mg	Fiber: 1.6 g	Sodium: 276 mg

Cajun Chicken Pasta

Yield: 4 servings

8 ounces linguine or fettuccine pasta

2 teaspoons crushed fresh garlic

8 ounces boneless skinless chicken
  breasts, cut into thin strips

1 pound fresh tomatoes, chopped
  (about 3 medium)

½ cup chopped onion

½ cup sliced celery (include leaves)

½ cup chopped green bell pepper

¼ cup unsalted tomato paste

1 teaspoon Cajun seasoning (or more
  to taste)

1 bay leaf

1. Cook the pasta al dente according to package directions. Drain well, return the pasta to the pot, and cover to keep warm.

2. While the pasta is cooking, coat a large nonstick skillet with nonstick cooking spray. Add the garlic and chicken, and stir-fry over medium-high heat for about 3 minutes, or until the chicken is browned.

3. Reduce the heat to low, and add all of the remaining ingredients except for the pasta to the skillet. Cover and simmer, stirring occasionally, for about 10 minutes, or until the vegetables are tender.

4. Add the pasta to the skillet mixture, and toss gently to mix. Remove the bay leaf and serve immediately.

NUTRITIONAL FACTS (PER 1½-CUP SERVING)

Calories: 324	Fat: 2.2 g	Protein: 22 g
Cholesterol: 33 mg	Fiber: 4 g	Sodium: 342 mg

Sonoma Spaghetti

Yield: 4 servings

½ cup chopped sun-dried tomatoes (not packed in oil)

½ cup water

8 ounces spaghetti or fettuccine pasta

1 cup nonfat or reduced-fat cream cheese

1 cup skim milk

¼ teaspoon ground white pepper

4 scallions, thinly sliced

2 tablespoons minced fresh basil

¼ cup grated nonfat or reduced-fat Parmesan cheese

1. Place the sun-dried tomatoes and water in a 1-quart saucepan, and bring to a boil over medium heat. Boil for 20 seconds, and remove the pot from the heat. Cover, and set aside for 20 minutes, or until the water has been absorbed.

2. Cook the pasta al dente according to package directions. Drain well, return the pasta to the pot, and cover to keep warm.

3. While the pasta is cooking, combine the cream cheese, milk, and pepper in a blender or food processor, and process until smooth. Pour the mixture into a 1-quart saucepan, and place over low heat. Cook and stir for about 2 minutes, or just until the sauce is heated through. Do not allow the sauce to boil. The sauce should be the consistency of heavy cream. Add a few tablespoons of skim milk, if necessary, to thin it to the desired consistency.

4. Drain any remaining liquid from the tomatoes, and add the tomatoes to the pasta. Add the sauce, scallions, and basil, and toss gently to mix. Serve immediately, topping each serving with a tablespoon of the Parmesan.

NUTRITIONAL FACTS (PER 1½-CUP SERVING)

Calories: 317	Fat: 1.2 g	Protein: 20.4 g
Cholesterol: 10 mg	Fiber: 2.4 g	Sodium: 493 mg

COOKING TIP

Cooking With Fresh Pasta

A variety of fresh pastas is now available in the refrigerated section of most grocery stores, and in some specialty shops, as well. Like their dry counterparts, most fresh pastas contain no added fat. To substitute fresh pasta for dry pastas in any of the recipes in this book, replace the required amount of dry pasta with 1¼ times as much fresh. For example, if a recipe calls for 8 ounces of linguini, substitute 10 ounces of fresh linguini. Fresh pasta cooks much faster than dry, so be sure to check the label for the recommended cooking time. Then enjoy the incomparable tenderness and delicacy of fresh pasta in a delicious low-fat dish.

Linguini With Clam Sauce

Yield: 4 servings

2 cans (6 ounces each) chopped clams, undrained

8 ounces linguine pasta

1 tablespoon olive oil (optional)

1 medium yellow onion, diced

1 cup sliced fresh mushrooms

½ cup thinly sliced celery (include leaves)

2 teaspoons crushed fresh garlic

¾ teaspoon dried basil

¾ teaspoon dried oregano

1 tablespoon butter-flavored sprinkles

⅛ teaspoon ground white pepper

¼ cup minced fresh parsley

⅓ cup grated nonfat or reduced-fat Parmesan cheese

1. Drain the clams, reserving ½ cup of the juice, and set aside.

2. Cook the pasta al dente according to package directions. Drain well, and return the pasta to the pot. If desired, add the olive oil and toss to mix. Cover the pot and set aside.

3. While the linguine is cooking, combine the onions, mushrooms, celery, garlic, basil, oregano, butter-flavored sprinkles, and pepper in a large skillet. Add the clams and the reserved juice, and bring to a boil over high heat. Reduce the heat to low, cover, and simmer, stirring occasionally, for 10 minutes, or until the vegetables are tender.

4. Add the cooked linguine and the parsley to the clam mixture, and toss gently until well mixed. Serve immediately, topping each serving with a rounded tablespoon of the Parmesan.

NUTRITIONAL FACTS (PER 1½-CUP SERVING)		
Calories: 318	Fat: 1.9 g	Protein: 22 g
Cholesterol: 36 mg	Fiber: 2.4 g	Sodium: 252 mg

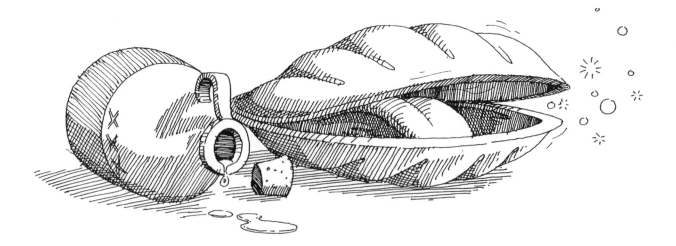

Spaghetti With Shrimp and Sun-Dried Tomatoes

1. Cook the pasta al dente according to package directions. Drain well, and return the pasta to the pot. If desired, add the olive oil and toss to mix. Cover the pot and set aside.

2. While the pasta is cooking, coat a large skillet with nonstick cooking spray. Add the garlic, shrimp, tomatoes, wine, broth, rosemary, and pepper to the skillet, and stir to mix. Cover and cook over medium heat for 3 minutes, or until the shrimp turn pink and the tomatoes plump. Reduce the heat to low.

3. Add the pasta to the shrimp mixture. Tossing gently, cook for a minute or 2, or until the mixture is heated through. Toss in the parsley, and serve immediately.

Yield: 4 servings

8 ounces thin spaghetti

1 tablespoon olive oil (optional)

2 teaspoons crushed fresh garlic

1 pound cleaned raw shrimp

½ cup diced sun-dried tomatoes (not packed in oil)

2 tablespoons dry white wine

½ cup chicken broth

1 teaspoon dried rosemary

¼ teaspoon ground black pepper

¼ cup minced fresh parsley

NUTRITIONAL FACTS (PER 1½-CUP SERVING)		
Calories: 318	Fat: 2.2 g	Protein: 27 g
Cholesterol: 166 mg	Fiber: 2.3 g	Sodium: 434 mg

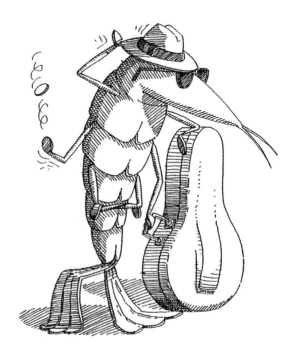

Getting the Fat Out of Your Pasta Recipes

It's a shame that most pasta recipes are so high in fat, as pasta is a natural for low-fat cooking. Happily, it's easy to do a healthy makeover of any pasta dish. Begin by leaving the oil—and the salt, too!—out of your cooking water. Pasta cooks up beautifully without this added fat. Then use the following table to replace high-fat foods like butter and sour cream with low- and no-fat ingredients.

Substitutions That Save Fat

Instead of:	Use:	You Save:	Special Considerations:
1 cup butter or margarine.	1 cup Butter Buds liquid.	1,500 calories, 176 fat grams.	Butter Buds may be used in sauces, but not for sautéing.
	1 cup reduced-fat margarine or light butter.	800–1,200 calories, 88–112 fat grams.	Nonfat margarines generally do not melt well enough to be used in cooking.
1 cup cream.	$\frac{2}{3}$ cup nonfat ricotta cheese blended with $\frac{1}{3}$ cup skim until smooth. (Add extra milk if the mixture is too thick.)	674 calories, 88 fat grams.	If using the ricotta mixture in a sauce that is to be heated, cook over low heat just until heated through. Some brands separate if boiled.
	1 cup evaporated skim milk.	622 calories, 88 fat grams.	Any of these substitutes may be used in cream sauces, casseroles, and other dishes.
	1 cup skim milk mixed with $\frac{1}{3}$ cup instant nonfat dry milk powder.	622 calories, 88 fat grams.	
1 cup sour cream.	1 cup nonfat sour cream.	252 calories, 48 fat grams.	Some brands of sour cream separate when heated. Choose a brand like Land O Lakes, which is heat stable, if the sour cream will be used in a cooked sauce.
	1 cup plain nonfat yogurt.	355 calories, 48 fat grams.	All yogurts will separate if heated. To prevent this, stir 2 tablespoons of flour or 1 tablespoon of cornstarch into each cup of yogurt before adding it to the sauce.
1 cup whole-milk ricotta cheese.	1 cup nonfat ricotta cheese.	248 calories, 32 fat grams.	This ingredient makes an excellent substitute in lasagna and other dishes.
1 cup regular cream cheese.	1 cup nonfat cream cheese.	600 calories, 80 fat grams.	If using nonfat cream cheese in a sauce that is to be heated, cook over low heat just until heated through. Some brands separate if boiled.
1 cup whole-milk mozzarella cheese.	1 cup nonfat mozzarella cheese.	200 calories, 28 fat grams.	This ingredient makes an excellent substitute in lasagna and other dishes.

Pasta With Crab and Asparagus

1. Combine all of the sauce ingredients in a blender or food processor, and process until smooth. Set aside.

2. Cook the pasta until almost al dente according to package directions. Add the asparagus to the cooking water, and cook for another minute, or until the asparagus are crisp-tender. Drain the pasta and asparagus, and return the mixture to the pot.

3. Add the crab meat to the pasta mixture, and top with the sauce. Place the pot over low heat, and, tossing gently, cook until the sauce is heated through. If the sauce is too thick, add a little skim milk.

4. Serve immediately, topping each serving with a tablespoon of the Parmesan.

Yield: 4 servings

8 ounces penne or sea shell pasta

½ pound fresh asparagus spears, cut into 1-inch pieces

6 ounces (about 1 cup) flaked cooked crab meat

¼ cup grated nonfat or reduced-fat Parmesan

SAUCE

1 cup nonfat ricotta cheese

2 scallions, chopped

2 tablespoons dry sherry

2 tablespoons lemon juice

¼ teaspoon dried oregano

⅛ teaspoon ground white pepper

NUTRITIONAL FACTS (PER 1½-CUP SERVING)		
Calories: 337	Fat: 1.6 g	Protein: 29 g
Cholesterol: 47 mg	Fiber: 2.7 g	Sodium: 332 mg

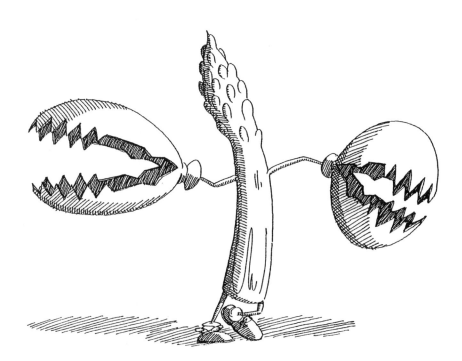

Bow Ties With Spicy Artichoke Sauce

Yield: 5 servings

8 ounces bow tie or rigatoni pasta

1 pound fresh tomatoes, diced (about 3 medium)

1 medium yellow onion, diced

1 cup sliced fresh mushrooms

1 tablespoon crushed fresh garlic

1 tablespoon dried basil

1 tablespoon dried oregano

¼ teaspoon cayenne pepper

¼ teaspoon ground black pepper

1 can (14 ounces) artichoke hearts, drained and quartered

½ red bell pepper, cut into thin strips

2 tablespoons lemon juice

½ cup plus 2 tablespoons grated nonfat or reduced-fat Parmesan cheese

1. Cook the pasta al dente according to package directions. Drain well, return the pasta to the pot, and cover to keep warm.

2. While the pasta is cooking, combine the tomatoes, onion, mushrooms, garlic, basil, oregano, cayenne, and black pepper in a large skillet. Place over medium-low heat, cover, and cook for 10 to 12 minutes, or until the tomatoes are soft.

3. Add the artichoke hearts, bell peppers, and lemon juice to the skillet mixture. Cover and cook for 2 additional minutes, or until the peppers are crisp-tender. Reduce the heat to low.

4. Add the pasta to the skillet mixture, and toss gently to mix. Add the Parmesan, toss gently, and serve immediately.

NUTRITIONAL FACTS (PER 1½-CUP SERVING)		
Calories: 235	Fat: 1.3 g	Protein: 13 g
Cholesterol: 6 mg	Fiber: 5.3 g	Sodium: 148 mg

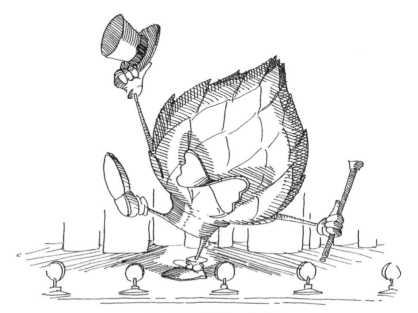

Pasta Primavera

Yield: 5 servings

1. Combine the cornstarch, pepper, and milk in a jar with a tight-fitting lid, and shake until the cornstarch has dissolved. Set aside.

2. Cook the pasta al dente according to package directions. Drain well, return the pasta to the pot, and cover to keep warm.

3. Coat a large skillet with nonstick cooking spray. Place over medium-high heat, add the garlic, and stir-fry for 30 seconds. Add the vegetables along with 1 tablespoon of water. Cover and cook, stirring occasionally, for 3 to 5 minutes, or until the vegetables are crisp-tender. Add a little more water if the skillet becomes too dry.

4. Reduce the heat to medium, and add the pasta to the skillet mixture. Shake the milk mixture, and add it to the skillet. Toss gently over medium heat for about 2 minutes, or just until the sauce begins to boil and thicken slightly.

5. Remove the skillet from the heat, and add the Parmesan. Toss gently to mix, and serve immediately.

2½ teaspoons cornstarch

¼ teaspoon ground white pepper

1½ cups evaporated skim milk

8 ounces spaghetti or fettuccine pasta

2 teaspoons crushed fresh garlic

½ cup thinly sliced carrots

½ cup sliced fresh mushrooms

2 cups fresh broccoli florets

½ small red bell pepper, cut into thin strips

1 medium onion, cut into thin wedges

½ cup plus 2 tablespoons grated nonfat or reduced-fat Parmesan cheese

NUTRITIONAL FACTS (PER 1½-CUP SERVING)

Calories: 291	Fat: 1.1 g	Protein: 17 g
Cholesterol: 10 mg	Fiber: 3.2 g	Sodium: 194 mg

Light and Lazy Lasagna

Yield: 10 servings

12 lasagna noodles

2 cups shredded nonfat or reduced-fat mozzarella cheese

¼ cup grated nonfat or reduced-fat Parmesan cheese

FILLING

15 ounces nonfat ricotta cheese

1 cup dry curd or nonfat cottage cheese

¼ cup grated nonfat or reduced-fat Parmesan cheese

2 tablespoons finely chopped fresh parsley, or 2 teaspoons dried

SAUCE

8 ounces 96% lean ground beef or turkey Italian sausage

2 cans (1 pound each) unsalted tomato sauce

1 can (1 pound) unsalted tomatoes, crushed

2 tablespoons tomato paste

2 cups sliced fresh mushrooms

1 medium onion, chopped

1½ teaspoons crushed fresh garlic

2½ teaspoons dried Italian seasoning

This lasagna is "lazy" because you don't cook the noodles before layering them in the pan. You can also prepare this entrée to the point of baking several hours—or even a day—in advance, and then refrigerate it until it's time to pop the dish into the oven.

1. To make the sauce, place the ground meat in a 4-quart pot. Cook over medium heat, stirring to crumble, until the meat is no longer pink. Drain off any fat. (If the meat is 96% lean, there will be no fat to drain.)

2. Add all of the remaining sauce ingredients to the browned meat, increase the heat to high, and bring to a boil. Reduce the heat to low, cover, and simmer for 25 minutes, or until the vegetables are tender. Set aside.

3. To make the filling, combine all of the filling ingredients in a large bowl, and stir to mix well. Set aside.

4. To assemble the lasagna, coat a 9-x-13-inch baking pan with nonstick cooking spray. Spoon 1 cup of the sauce over the bottom of the pan. Lay 4 of the uncooked noodles over the bottom of the pan, arranging 3 of the noodles lengthwise and 1 noodle crosswise. Allow a little space between the noodles for expansion. (You will have to break 1 inch off the crosswise noodle to make it fit in the pan.)

5. Top the noodles with half of the filling mixture, ¾ cup of the mozzarella, and 1½ cups of the sauce. Repeat the noodles, filling, mozzarella, and sauce layers. Finally, top with the remaining noodles, sauce, Parmesan, and mozzarella.

6. Cover the pan with aluminum foil, and bake at 350°F for 45 minutes. Remove the foil, and bake for 15 additional minutes, or until the edges are bubbly and the top is browned. Remove the dish from the oven, and let sit for 5 minutes before cutting and serving.

NUTRITIONAL FACTS (PER SERVING)

Calories: 288	Fat: 1.7 g	Protein: 28 g
Cholesterol: 27 mg	Fiber: 3 g	Sodium: 367 mg

Lasagna Roll-Ups

1. To make the sauce, combine all of the sauce ingredients in a 1½-quart pot, and bring to a boil over medium-high heat. Reduce the heat to low, cover, and simmer for 20 minutes.

2. To make the filling, combine all of the filling ingredients in a medium-sized bowl, and stir to mix well. Set aside.

3. Cook the noodles al dente according to package directions. Drain, rinse, and drain again.

4. Coat a 2½-quart casserole dish with nonstick cooking spray. To assemble the roll-ups, arrange the noodles on a flat surface, and spread ⅛ of the filling mixture along the length of each noodle. Roll each noodle up jelly-roll style, and place in the prepared dish, seam side down. Pour the sauce over the roll-ups.

5. Cover the dish with aluminum foil, and bake at 350°F for 30 minutes. Remove the foil, top with the mozzarella, and bake for 10 additional minutes, or until the cheese is melted. Serve hot.

NUTRITIONAL FACTS (PER SERVING)		
Calories: 384	Fat: 1.4 g	Protein: 35 g
Cholesterol: 22 mg	Fiber: 6.0 g	Sodium: 412 mg

Time-Saving Tip

In a hurry? Instead of preparing homemade sauce for your Lasagna Roll-Ups, use 3 cups of bottled fat-free marinara sauce.

Yield: 4 servings

8 lasagna noodles

1 cup shredded nonfat or reduced-fat mozzarella cheese

FILLING

15 ounces nonfat ricotta cheese

1 package (10 ounces) frozen chopped spinach, thawed and squeezed dry

½ cup grated carrot

2 tablespoons minced fresh parsley

SAUCE

1 can (1 pound) unsalted tomatoes, crushed

1 can (6 ounces) unsalted tomato paste

¼ cup unsalted vegetable broth or water

1 medium yellow onion, chopped

1 teaspoon dried Italian seasoning

1 teaspoon crushed fresh garlic

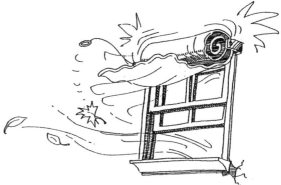

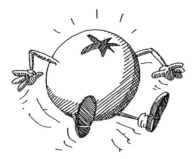

Florentine Stuffed Shells

Yield: 8 servings

24 jumbo pasta shells

FILLING

15 ounces nonfat ricotta cheese

½ cup shredded nonfat or
  reduced-fat mozzarella cheese

¼ cup grated nonfat or reduced-fat
  Parmesan cheese

1 package (10 ounces) frozen
  chopped spinach or broccoli,
  thawed and squeezed dry

¼ cup finely chopped onion

½ teaspoon dried Italian seasoning

SAUCE

1 can (1 pound) unsalted tomatoes,
  crushed

1 can (6 ounces) tomato paste

½ cup finely chopped onion

1 teaspoon crushed fresh garlic

¼ cup dry red wine, beef broth, or
  vegetable broth

2 tablespoons grated nonfat or
  reduced-fat Parmesan cheese

2 teaspoons dried Italian seasoning

¼ teaspoon ground black pepper

1. To make the sauce, combine all of the sauce ingredients in a 1½-quart pot, and bring to a boil over medium-high heat. Reduce the heat to low, cover, and simmer for 20 minutes.

2. To make the filling, combine all of the filling ingredients in a medium-sized bowl, and stir to mix well. Set aside.

3. Cook the pasta al dente according to package directions. Drain, rinse, and drain again. Set aside.

4. To assemble the dish, coat a 9-x-13-inch baking pan with nonstick cooking spray. Spoon 1 rounded tablespoon of the filling into each shell, and arrange the stuffed shells in a single layer in the pan. Pour the sauce over the shells.

5. Bake at 350°F for 25 to 30 minutes, or until heated through. Serve hot.

NUTRITIONAL FACTS (PER SERVING)		
Calories: 257	Fat: 1.1 g	Protein: 18 g
Cholesterol: 9 mg	Fiber: 3.6 g	Sodium: 361 mg

Time-Saving Tip

To speed preparation, make Florentine Stuffed Shells with 3 cups of bottled fat-free marinara sauce instead of the homemade sauce.

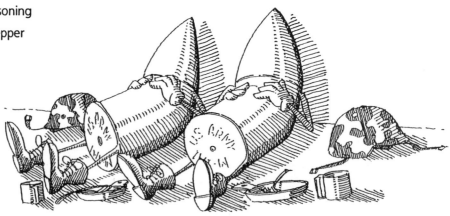

9. Hearty Home-Style Entrées

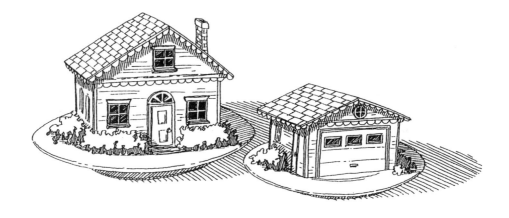

Many people believe that a transition to low-fat cooking means waving good-bye to the hearty home-style dishes they love so much. The truth is that you don't have to give up pot roast with gravy, chicken and dumplings, shepherd's pie, or any of your other favorites just because you're cutting down on fat. Nor do you have to spend hours in specialty stores searching for exotic ingredients, or added time in the kitchen learning complicated cooking methods. By replacing high-fat ingredients with low-fat or no-fat foods, and by using a few simple cooking techniques, you can enjoy all of your favorite foods and many new ones, as well. This chapter will show you how.

The entrées in this chapter begin with the freshest seafood or the leanest cuts of poultry, beef, or pork. Then, fat is kept to an absolute mininum by using nonstick skillets and nonstick cooking sprays, and by replacing full-fat dairy products with their healthful nonfat and reduced-fat counterparts. Of course, fresh vegetables, hearty grains, and savory seasonings play an important role in these dishes by adding their own great flavors and textures, and by boosting nutrition. The result? Satisfying home-style entrées, most of which have only 2 to 3 grams of fat per serving!

As you glance through the pages of this chapter, remember that these are just *some* of the delicious low-fat entrées that are within your reach. Delicious pasta entrées are presented in Chapter 8, and crowd-pleasing meatless main dishes can be found in Chapter 10. And, of course, many of your own family favorites can be easily "slimmed down" with the techniques and ingredients used within this chapter. Spicy jambalayas, "fried" chicken, juicy burgers, and more can all be part of a healthy diet once you learn the secrets of fat-free cooking!

Lemon-Herb Chicken With Vegetables

Yield: 4 servings

4 boneless skinless chicken breast halves (4 ounces each)

¼ cup chicken broth

16 medium whole fresh mushrooms (about 8 ounces)

2 medium carrots, peeled, halved lengthwise, and cut into 2-inch pieces

2 medium zucchini, halved lengthwise and cut into ½-inch slices

MARINADE

2 tablespoons lemon juice

1 tablespoon brown sugar

1 teaspoon crushed fresh garlic

½ teaspoon coarsely ground black pepper

¼ teaspoon salt

1 teaspoon dried thyme, oregano, or rosemary

1. Rinse the chicken, and pat it dry with paper towels. Place the chicken in a shallow nonmetal container.

2. Combine the marinade ingredients in a small bowl, and pour over the chicken parts. Turn the chicken to coat, cover, and refrigerate for several hours or overnight.

3. Coat a large skillet with nonstick cooking spray, and preheat over medium-high heat. Place the chicken in the skillet, reserving the marinade, and cook for about 2 minutes on each side, or until nicely browned.

4. Reduce the heat to low, and add the reserved marinade, broth, mushrooms, and carrots to the skillet. Cover and simmer for 10 minutes. Add the zucchini, and simmer for an additional 5 minutes, or until the chicken is no longer pink inside and the vegetables are tender.

5. Serve hot, accompanying each chicken breast with some of the vegetables and pan juices. Serve over brown rice if desired.

NUTRITIONAL FACTS (PER SERVING)		
Calories: 192	Fat: 3.4 g	Protein: 29 g
Cholesterol: 72 mg	Fiber: 2.7 g	Sodium: 263 mg

FAT-FREE COOKING TIP

Browning Without Fat

The traditional method of browning foods requires oil, butter, or margarine. Indeed, some recipes recommend several tablespoons of oil for browning! However, as the recipes in this chapter show, all that extra oil is simply not necessary. To brown meat, chicken, or vegetables with virtually no added fat, spray a thin film of nonstick cooking spray over the bottom of the skillet. Then preheat the skillet over medium-high heat, and brown the food as usual. If the food starts to stick, add a few teaspoons of water or broth. If you use a nonstick skillet *and* nonstick cooking spray, it should not be necessary to add any liquid at all.

.hicken With Garlic n-Dried Tomatoes

As ... *sweet and mild. For a real*
tre... *h bread instead of butter.*

1. ... ' with paper towels.

2 ... with olive oil cooking spray,
... t. Crush 2 of the garlic cloves,
... the chicken in the skillet, and
an... s around the chicken.

3. ... minutes on each side, or until
the chicken and ga... e nicely browned. Remove the
chicken from the skillet, and set aside. Remove the skillet from
the heat.

4. Lay the onions and tomatoes over the garlic cloves in the
skillet. Arrange the chicken in a single layer over the tomatoes,
onions, and garlic. Pour the wine and broth over the chicken, and
sprinkle with the oregano and pepper.

5. Cover and bake at 350°F for 30 minutes, or until the chicken
is tender and the juices run clear when the chicken is pierced.

6. Serve hot, accompanying each chicken breast with some of
the vegetables and pan juices. Serve over brown rice or noodles
if desired.

4 boneless skinless chicken breast
halves (4 ounces each)

20 cloves garlic, peeled (about 2 heads)

1 medium onion, sliced ¼-inch-thick
and separated into rings

½ cup chopped sun-dried tomatoes
(not packed in oil)

¼ cup dry white wine

½ cup chicken broth

1 teaspoon dried oregano

¼ teaspoon ground black pepper

NUTRITIONAL FACTS (PER SERVING)		
Calories: 209	Fat: 3.3 g	Protein: 30 g
Cholesterol: 72 mg	Fiber: 1.7 g	Sodium: 305 mg

Poached Chicken
With Creamy Mushroom Sauce

Yield: 4 servings

4 boneless skinless chicken breast halves (4 ounces each)

1 cup chicken broth

SAUCE

2 cups sliced fresh mushrooms

¾ cup nonfat sour cream

1 tablespoon unbleached flour

¼ teaspoon ground black pepper

1 tablespoon freshly grated lemon rind

1. Rinse the chicken, and arrange it in an unheated nonstick skillet. Add the broth, and bring to a boil over high heat. Reduce the heat to low, cover, and simmer for 20 to 25 minutes, or until the chicken is tender and no longer pink inside. Pour the broth into a measuring cup. Transfer the chicken to a serving platter, and cover to keep warm.

2. To make the sauce, place the mushrooms in the skillet along with 1 tablespoon of the reserved broth. Cook and stir over medium heat until the mushrooms are tender and all of the liquid has evaporated. Add ½ cup plus 2 tablespoons of the reserved broth, and bring to a boil. Reduce the heat to medium-low.

3. Combine the sour cream, flour, pepper, and lemon rind in a small bowl, and stir until smooth. Add the sour cream mixture to the mushroom mixture, and cook and stir for about 1 minute, or until the sauce is thickened and bubbly.

4. Pour the sauce over the chicken, and serve hot, accompanying the dish with brown rice or noodles if desired.

NUTRITIONAL FACTS (PER SERVING)		
Calories: 207	Fat: 3.2 g	Protein: 30 g
Cholesterol: 72 mg	Fiber: 0.5 g	Sodium: 231 mg

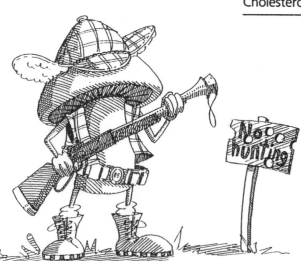

Chicken With Black Bean Salsa

Yield: 6 servings

1. Rinse the chicken, and pat it dry with paper towels. Spread each piece with some of the garlic, and sprinkle with the pepper.

2. Coat a large skillet with nonstick cooking spray, and preheat over medium-high heat. Arrange the chicken in the skillet, and cook for about 2 minutes on each side, or until nicely browned. Reduce the heat to low, and add the broth. Cover and simmer for 10 to 12 minutes, or until the chicken is tender and the juices run clear when the chicken is pierced. Transfer the chicken to a serving platter, and cover to keep warm.

3. Drain any liquid from the skillet, and add the undrained black beans and the salsa or picante sauce. Cook and stir over medium heat until heated through. Spoon the bean mixture over the chicken, sprinkle with the scallions, and serve hot, accompanying the dish with brown rice if desired.

6 boneless skinless chicken breast halves (4 ounces each)

1 tablespoon crushed fresh garlic

¼ teaspoon ground black pepper

3 tablespoons chicken broth

1 can (15 ounces) black beans, undrained

½ cup salsa or picante sauce

3 tablespoons thinly sliced scallions

NUTRITIONAL FACTS (PER SERVING)		
Calories: 212	Fat: 3.4 g	Protein: 30 g
Cholesterol: 72 mg	Fiber: 4.9 g	Sodium: 436 mg

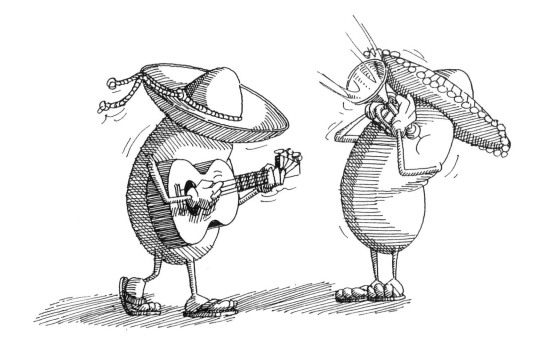

Crispy Cajun Chicken

Yield: 8 servings

8 skinless chicken breast halves with bones (6 ounces each)

1¼ cups nonfat buttermilk or yogurt

COATING

5 cups corn flakes

1 tablespoon ground paprika

2–3 teaspoons Cajun seasoning

Finely crushed corn flakes give this ultra-lean oven-fried chicken its crispy coating.

1. Rinse the chicken, and pat it dry with paper towels. Place the chicken in a shallow nonmetal dish, and pour the buttermilk or yogurt over the chicken. Turn the pieces to coat, cover, and refrigerate for several hours or overnight.

2. To make the coating, place the corn flakes in a blender or food processor, and process into crumbs. You should have about 1¼ cups of crumbs. (Adjust the amount if necessary.)

3. Combine the corn flake crumbs, paprika, and Cajun seasoning in a small plastic bag. Close the bag, and shake well to mix.

4. Remove 2 pieces of chicken from the buttermilk, place in the coating bag, and shake to coat evenly. Repeat with the remaining chicken.

5. Coat a large baking sheet with nonstick cooking spray, and arrange the chicken on the pan. Lightly spray each piece of chicken with nonstick cooking spray, and bake at 400°F for 50 minutes, or until the meat is tender and the juices run clear when the chicken is pierced. Serve hot.

NUTRITIONAL FACTS (PER SERVING)

Calories: 207	Fat: 3.2 g	Protein: 28 g
Cholesterol: 72 mg	Fiber: 0.4 g	Sodium: 285 mg

Simply Delicious Chicken and Dumplings

1. Rinse the chicken, and place the chicken, water, bouillon granules, poultry seasoning, and pepper in a 4-quart pot. Bring the mixture to a boil over high heat. Then reduce the heat to low, cover, and simmer for 25 to 30 minutes, or until the chicken is tender and the juices run clear when the chicken is pierced.

2. Remove the pot from the heat. Remove the chicken from the pot with a slotted spoon, reserving the liquid. Arrange the chicken on a plate to cool slightly.

3. Pour the cooking liquid into a fat separator cup, and pour the fat-free broth from the separator cup into a measuring cup. There should be 3 cups. (If necessary, add water to bring it up to measure.) Return the broth to the pot.

4. Remove the skin and bones from the chicken, and discard. Tear the remaining meat into bite-sized pieces, and return the chicken to the pot.

5. Add the carrots, celery, and onion to the pot. Place the pot over high heat, and bring to a boil. Reduce the heat to low, cover, and simmer for 5 minutes, or until the vegetables are almost tender. Add the peas to the pot.

6. Combine the milk and flour in a jar with a tight-fitting lid, and shake until smooth. Pour the flour mixture into the pot, and cook, stirring constantly, for about 2 minutes, or until the broth is thickened and bubbly.

7. To make the dumplings, combine the flour, baking powder, and sugar in a medium-sized bowl, and stir to mix well. Stir in the buttermilk, and drop heaping teaspoonfuls of the batter onto the simmering stew. Cover and simmer over low heat for 10 to 12 minutes, or until the dumplings are fluffy and cooked through. Serve hot.

Yield: 6 servings

4 chicken breast halves with skin and bone (8 ounces each)

2½ cups water

1½ teaspoons chicken bouillon granules

½ teaspoon poultry seasoning

⅛ teaspoon ground white pepper

1 medium carrot, peeled, halved lengthwise, and sliced

1 stalk celery, thinly sliced (include leaves)

½ cup chopped onion

1 cup frozen green peas

½ cup skim milk

¼ cup plus 2 tablespoons unbleached flour

DUMPLINGS

1½ cups unbleached flour

2 teaspoons baking powder

1 teaspoon sugar

¾ cup nonfat buttermilk

NUTRITIONAL FACTS (PER 1½-CUP SERVING)

Calories: 257	Fat: 1.8 g	Protein: 24 g
Cholesterol: 45 mg	Fiber: 2.9 g	Sodium: 498 mg

Chicken Enchiladas

Yield: 6 servings

1¼ pounds boneless skinless chicken breasts

2 cups water

1 teaspoon chicken bouillon granules

⅓ cup thinly sliced scallions

¼ cup minced fresh cilantro or parsley

1 teaspoon dried oregano

¼ teaspoon ground black pepper

12 corn tortillas (6-inch rounds)

1 cup shredded nonfat or reduced-fat Cheddar cheese

SAUCE

1 can (8 ounces) unsalted tomato sauce

1½ tablespoons chili powder

1½ teaspoons ground cumin

2 tablespoons unbleached flour

¼ cup water

TOPPINGS

¾ cup nonfat sour cream

¼ cup thinly sliced scallions

NUTRITIONAL FACTS
(PER 2-ENCHILADA SERVING)

Calories: 318	Fiber: 3.7 g
Chol: 58 mg	Protein: 32 g
Fat: 2.8 g	Sodium: 449 mg

Softening the tortillas in tomato sauce instead of the usual oil or lard saves lots of fat and calories, as does using nonfat cheese and skinless chicken breasts.

1. Rinse the chicken, and place the chicken, water, and bouillon granules in a 2-quart pot. Bring the mixture to a boil over high heat. Then reduce the heat to low, cover, and simmer for 20 minutes, or until the chicken is tender and the juices run clear when the chicken is pierced.

2. Remove the chicken from the pot with a slotted spoon, reserving the liquid, and cool to room temperature. Tear the chicken into shreds, and transfer to a large bowl. Add the scallions, cilantro or parsley, oregano, and pepper, and stir to mix. Set aside.

3. To make the sauce, combine the tomato sauce, chili powder, and cumin in a medium-sized skillet. Stir in 1½ cups of the reserved cooking liquid, and bring the mixture to a boil over medium heat.

4. Combine the flour and water in a jar with a tight-fitting lid, and shake until smooth. Stir the flour mixture into the simmering sauce, and continue to stir until the mixture is thickened and bubbly. Reduce the heat to low.

5. Coat a 9-x-13-inch baking pan with nonstick cooking spray. Dip a tortilla in the sauce for about 10 seconds—just long enough to soften the tortilla—coating each side with sauce. Lay the tortilla on a flat surface, and place ¼ cup of the chicken filling along one end. Roll the tortilla up jelly-roll style, and lay it in the pan, seam side down. Repeat with the remaining tortillas, leaving a ¼-inch space between the enchiladas to prevent them from sticking together.

6. Pour the remaining sauce over the enchiladas, and spread the cheese over the top. Bake uncovered at 450°F for 12 to 15 minutes, or until the cheese is melted and the dish is heated through. Top individual servings with 2 tablespoons of sour cream and 2 teaspoons of scallions, and serve hot.

Savory Turkey and Rice

1. Rinse the turkey, and pat it dry with paper towels. Coat a 9-inch square pan with nonstick cooking spray, and arrange the turkey in a single layer in the pan. Add 2 tablespoons of the broth or water, cover with aluminum foil, and bake at 350°F for 20 minutes. Remove the foil, and bake for 10 additional minutes, or until the meat is tender and the juices run clear when the turkey is pierced.

2. Remove the turkey from the pan, and cool to room temperature. Tear the meat into bite-sized pieces, and set aside.

3. Combine the rice, $4\frac{1}{2}$ cups of the broth or water, and the bouillon granules in a $2\frac{1}{2}$-quart pot. Bring the mixture to a boil over high heat, stir, and reduce the heat to low. Cover and simmer without stirring for 45 to 50 minutes, or until the liquid has been absorbed and the rice is tender. Remove the pot from the heat, and allow to sit, covered, for 5 minutes.

4. Combine the mushrooms, onion, garlic, poultry seasoning, pepper, and sherry in a large nonstick skillet. Sauté over medium heat until the mushrooms are tender and most of the liquid has evaporated. Add the peas, rice, turkey, and remaining $\frac{1}{4}$ cup of broth or water, and toss until heated through. Serve hot.

1 pound turkey breast tenderloins

$4\frac{3}{4}$ cups plus 2 tablespoons unsalted chicken broth or water, divided

2 cups uncooked brown rice

2 teaspoons chicken bouillon granules

$1\frac{1}{4}$ cups sliced fresh mushrooms

1 medium yellow onion, chopped

1 teaspoon crushed fresh garlic

$\frac{3}{4}$ teaspoon poultry seasoning

$\frac{1}{4}$ teaspoon ground black pepper

2 tablespoons dry sherry

1 cup frozen green peas, thawed

NUTRITIONAL FACTS (PER $1\frac{1}{2}$-CUP SERVING)

Calories: 341	Fat: 2.8 g	Protein: 24 g
Cholesterol: 49 mg	Fiber: 3.8 g	Sodium: 403 mg

Breast of Turkey Provençal

Yield: 4 servings

4 pieces (4 ounces each) turkey breast tenderloins or turkey cutlets

⅓ cup unbleached flour

¼ teaspoon salt

¼ teaspoon ground black pepper

½ cup dry white wine

2 teaspoons crushed fresh garlic

1 teaspoon dried rosemary

1 teaspoon dried oregano

1 bay leaf

½ cup chicken broth

1 medium tomato, cut into 8 wedges

¼ cup minced fresh parsley

1. Rinse the turkey, and pat it dry with paper towels. Place the turkey on a flat surface, and pound to ¼-inch thickness.

2. Combine the flour, salt, and pepper in a plastic bag. Close the bag, and shake well to mix. Place the turkey, 2 pieces at a time, in the coating bag, and shake well until evenly coated. Set aside.

3. Combine the wine, garlic, rosemary, and oregano in a small bowl. Set aside.

4. Coat a large nonstick skillet with olive oil cooking spray, and preheat over medium-high heat. Add the turkey, and cook for 2 to 3 minutes on each side, or until nicely browned.

5. Pour the wine mixture over the turkey, and add the bay leaf. Reduce the heat to medium-low, and cook until the wine is reduced by half, periodically scraping the bottom of the skillet. Add the chicken broth, and arrange the tomato wedges around the meat. Cover and simmer for 5 to 7 minutes, or until the turkey and tomatoes are tender.

6. Transfer the turkey, vegetables, and sauce to a serving platter, and sprinkle with the parsley. Serve over noodles or pasta if desired.

NUTRITIONAL FACTS (PER SERVING)		
Calories: 177	Fat: 1.5 g	Protein: 28 g
Cholesterol: 73 mg	Fiber: 0.8 g	Sodium: 283 mg

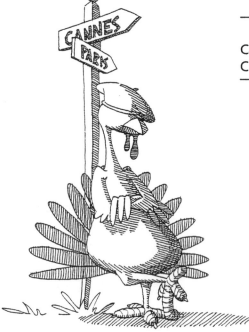

Turkey Jambalaya

For variety, make this savory dish with chicken instead of turkey.

1. Rinse the turkey, and pat it dry with paper towels. Coat a large skillet with nonstick cooking spray, and preheat over medium-high heat. Add the turkey, and stir-fry for 2 to 3 minutes, or until browned.

2. Add the remaining ingredients to the skillet, and stir to mix well. Bring the mixture to a boil, reduce the heat to low, and cover. Simmer for about 50 minutes, or until the liquid has been absorbed and the rice is tender.

3. Remove the skillet from the heat, and allow to sit, covered, for 5 minutes. Serve hot.

Yield: 5 servings

¾ pound boneless skinless turkey breasts, cut into bite-sized pieces

1⅔ cups unsalted chicken broth

1½ cups uncooked brown rice

4 ounces smoked turkey sausage (at least 97% lean), diced

1 can (1 pound) unsalted tomatoes, crushed

½ cup thinly sliced celery (include leaves)

½ cup chopped green bell pepper

½ cup chopped onion

1 teaspoon crushed fresh garlic

1 bay leaf

1–2 teaspoons Cajun or Creole seasoning

NUTRITIONAL FACTS (PER 1½-CUP SERVING)

Calories: 340	Fat: 3.5 g	Protein: 25 g
Cholesterol: 56 mg	Fiber: 3.5 g	Sodium: 386 mg

Mexican Skillet Dinner

1. Place the meat in a large, deep skillet, and cook over medium heat, stirring to crumble, until the meat is no longer pink. Add all of the remaining ingredients, and stir to mix well.

2. Bring the mixture to a boil. Then reduce the heat to low, cover, and simmer, stirring occasionally, for 10 to 12 minutes, or until the pasta is tender and the liquid has been absorbed. If any liquid remains, remove the cover and simmer for several more minutes. Serve hot.

Yield: 6 servings

1 pound 96% lean ground beef

1 can (1 pound) Mexican-style tomatoes, crushed

2½ cups fresh or frozen (thawed) whole kernel corn

1 teaspoon crushed fresh garlic

8 ounces whole wheat macaroni

1⅓ cups unsalted beef broth or water

1 tablespoon chili powder

½ teaspoon dried oregano

¼ teaspoon ground black pepper

½ teaspoon salt (optional)

NUTRITIONAL FACTS (PER 1½-CUP SERVING)

Calories: 278	Fat: 3.3 g	Protein: 22 g
Cholesterol: 40 mg	Fiber: 6 g	Sodium: 378 mg

Foil-Baked Flounder

Yield: 4 servings

4 flounder, sole, snapper, or orange
   roughy fillets (6 ounces each)

2 teaspoons crushed fresh garlic

2 cups snow peas

2 cups thinly sliced carrots (about 2
   medium)

¼ cup chopped scallions

2 tablespoons plus 2 teaspoons
   minced fresh dill

2 teaspoons butter-flavored sprinkles

½ teaspoon ground black pepper

¼ cup dry white wine

Baking fish in a foil pouch allows the fish to steam in its own juices, sealing in flavor and nutrients. Vegetables, wine, and herbs—not fat or salt—provide added flavor and color.

1. Cut heavy-duty aluminum foil into four 8-x-12-inch pieces, and center a fish fillet on the lower half of each piece. Spread ½ teaspoon of garlic over each fillet, and top with ½ cup of snow peas, ½ cup of carrots, 1 tablespoon of scallions, 2 teaspoons of dill, ½ teaspoon of butter sprinkles, ⅛ teaspoon of pepper, and 1 tablespoon of wine.

2. Fold the upper half of the foil over the fish to meet the bottom half. Seal the edges together by making a tight ½-inch fold; then fold again to double-seal. Allow space for heat circulation and expansion. Use this technique to seal the remaining sides.

3. Arrange the pouches on a baking pan or directly on the oven rack, and bake at 450°F for about 15 minutes, or until the fish is opaque and the thickest part is easily flaked with a fork. Open each packet by cutting an "X" in the top of the foil, and serve hot.

NUTRITIONAL FACTS (PER SERVING)

Calories: 223	Fat: 2.3 g	Protein: 35 g
Cholesterol: 82 mg	Fiber: 3.2 g	Sodium: 176 mg

Spicy Shrimp Gumbo

1. Combine the onion, bell pepper, celery, garlic, sausage, tomato sauce, broth, bay leaf, and Cajun or Creole seasoning in a $2\frac{1}{2}$-quart pot, and bring to a boil over high heat. Reduce the heat to low, cover, and simmer for 20 minutes, or until the vegetables are tender.

2. Add the corn and okra to the sausage mixture. Increase the heat to high, and bring to a boil. Then reduce the heat to low, cover, and simmer for 5 minutes, or until the okra is barely tender.

3. Add the shrimp to the gumbo, cover, and simmer for 5 additional minutes, or until the shrimp turn pink. Serve hot, accompanying the dish with brown rice, if desired.

NUTRITIONAL FACTS (PER 1-CUP SERVING)

Calories: 134	Fat: 1.1 g	Protein: 14.5 g
Cholesterol: 91 mg	Fiber: 3.2 g	Sodium: 357 mg

Yield: 6 cups

1 medium onion, chopped

1 medium green bell pepper, chopped

$\frac{1}{2}$ cup thinly sliced celery (include leaves)

2 teaspoons crushed fresh garlic

4 ounces smoked turkey sausage (at least 97% lean), diced

1 can (1 pound) unsalted tomato sauce

$\frac{1}{2}$ cup unsalted chicken broth

1 bay leaf

1 teaspoon Cajun or Creole seasoning (or more to taste)

1 cup frozen whole kernel corn

1 cup frozen cut okra

$\frac{3}{4}$ pound cleaned raw shrimp

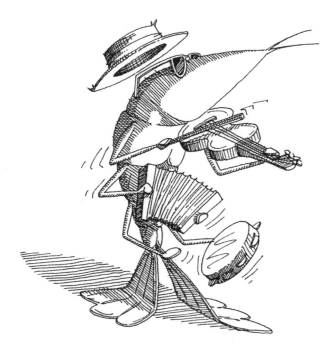

Pot Roast With Sour Cream Gravy

Yield: 8 servings

2½-pound top round roast or London broil

2 teaspoons crushed fresh garlic

¼ teaspoon coarsely ground black pepper

1 medium yellow onion, thinly sliced

2 bay leaves

¾ cup beef broth

1½ pounds potatoes (about 5 medium), scrubbed and quartered

1¼ pounds carrots (about 6 large), peeled and cut into 2-inch pieces

GRAVY

Meat drippings

1½ teaspoons beef bouillon granules

3 tablespoons unbleached flour

¼ cup water

½ cup nonfat sour cream

NUTRITIONAL FACTS
(PER SERVING)

Calories: 300	Fiber: 4.2 g
Chol: 59 mg	Protein: 29 g
Fat: 5.2 g	Sodium: 335 mg

Top round roast—which is sometimes sold as London broil—is one of the leanest cuts available, and can be easily substituted for pot roasts and briskets in any of your favorite recipes.

1. Trim any visible fat from the meat. Rinse the meat, and pat it dry with paper towels. Spread the garlic over both sides of the meat, and sprinkle with the pepper.

2. Coat a large ovenproof skillet with nonstick cooking spray, and preheat over medium-high heat. Place the meat in the skillet, and brown for 2 to 3 minutes on each side. Remove the skillet from the heat, and spread the onions over the meat. Place the bay leaves in the skillet, and pour the broth into the bottom of the skillet. Cover tightly, and bake at 325°F for 1 hour and 45 minutes.

3. Remove the skillet from the oven, and carefully remove the cover. (Steam will escape.) Place the potatoes and carrots around the meat, cover, and return the skillet to the oven for 45 additional minutes, or until the meat and vegetables are tender. Transfer the meat and vegetables to a serving platter, and cover to keep warm.

4. To make the gravy, discard the bay leaves, and pour the meat drippings into a fat separator cup. Then pour the fat-free drippings into a 2-cup measure. (If the meat was well trimmed, there may not be any fat to remove.) If necessary, add water to the defatted drippings to bring the volume up to 1¼ cups.

5. Pour the drippings mixture into a 1-quart saucepan, add the bouillon granules, and bring to a boil over medium heat. Combine the flour and water in a jar with a tight-fitting lid, and shake until smooth. Slowly pour the flour mixture into the boiling gravy. Cook and stir with a wire whisk until the gravy is thickened and bubbly.

6. Reduce the heat to low, add the sour cream, and whisk just until heated through. Transfer the gravy to a warmed gravy boat or pitcher, and serve hot with the meat and vegetables.

Italian-Style Pot Roast

1. Trim any visible fat from the meat. Rinse the meat, and pat it dry with paper towels. Spread the garlic over both sides of the meat, and sprinkle with the pepper.

2. Coat a large ovenproof skillet with nonstick cooking spray, and preheat over medium-high heat. Place the meat in the skillet, and brown for 2 to 3 minutes on each side. Remove the skillet from the heat, and spread the onions and mushrooms over the meat. Combine the tomatoes, tomato paste, water, Italian seasoning, and bouillion granules in a large bowl, and pour over the meat and vegetables.

3. Cover tightly, and bake at 350°F for 2 hours, or until the meat is tender. Serve hot, accompanying the roast with spaghetti, linguini, or another pasta if desired.

Yield: 6 servings

1¾-pound top round roast or London broil

2 teaspoons crushed fresh garlic

¼ teaspoon ground black pepper

1 cup chopped onion

1½ cups sliced fresh mushrooms

1 can (1 pound) unsalted tomatoes, crushed

1 can (6 ounces) unsalted tomato paste

¼ cup water

2 teaspoons dried Italian seasoning

1¾ teaspoons beef bouillon granules

NUTRITIONAL FACTS (PER SERVING)		
Calories: 205	Fat: 5 g	Protein: 27 g
Cholesterol: 59 mg	Fiber: 3.3 g	Sodium: 336 mg

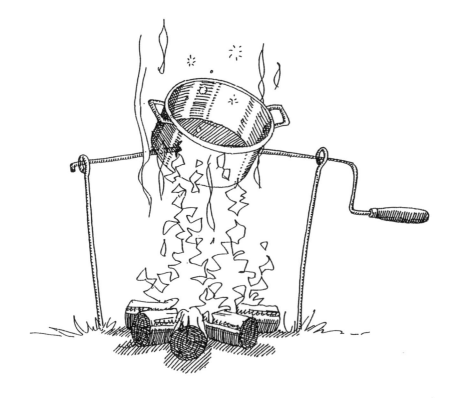

Old-Fashioned Beef Stew

Yield: 8 cups

1 pound top round

1 can (1 pound) unsalted tomato sauce

2 cups water

¼ teaspoon ground black pepper

1 teaspoon dried thyme

1 teaspoon dried marjoram

2 bay leaves

1½ teaspoons beef bouillon granules

1 tablespoon Worcestershire sauce

2 medium potatoes, scrubbed and diced

2 medium carrots, peeled, halved, and sliced

1 medium yellow onion, diced

1 cup sliced fresh mushrooms

1 medium stalk celery, thinly sliced (include leaves)

1 cup frozen green peas, thawed

1. Trim any visible fat from the meat. Rinse the meat, and pat it dry with paper towels. Cut the meat into bite-sized pieces.

2. Coat a large deep skillet or Dutch oven with nonstick cooking spray, and preheat over medium-high heat. Add the meat, and brown for 2 to 3 minutes.

3. Stir the tomato sauce, water, pepper, herbs, bouillon granules, and Worcestershire sauce into the meat, and bring to a boil. Reduce the heat to low, cover, and simmer for 1 hour, or until the meat is tender.

4. Add the potatoes, carrots, onion, mushrooms, and celery to the meat. Cover and simmer for 30 minutes, or until the vegetables are tender. Add the peas, and simmer for 10 additional minutes. Serve hot.

NUTRITIONAL FACTS (PER 1-CUP SERVING)		
Calories: 165	Fat: 2.6 g	Protein: 16 g
Cholesterol: 29 mg	Fiber: 3.4 g	Sodium: 285 mg

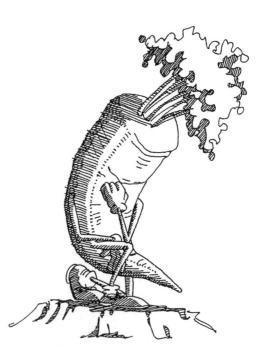

Mama Mia Meat Loaf

"Lean" meat loaf pans are great for low-fat cooking. These pans have an inner liner with holes in it that allows the fat to drain into the bottom of the pan instead of being reabsorbed into the meat.

1. Combine the loaf ingredients in a large bowl, and mix well. Coat a 9-x-5-inch meat loaf pan with nonstick cooking spray, and press the mixture into the pan to form a loaf.

2. Bake uncovered at 350°F for 35 minutes. Combine the topping ingredients in a small bowl, and pour the topping over the meat loaf. Bake for 30 additional minutes, or until the meat is no longer pink inside. Remove the loaf from the oven, and let sit for 10 minutes before slicing and serving.

NUTRITIONAL FACTS (PER SERVING)

Calories: 142	Fat: 3.7 g	Protein: 19 g
Cholesterol: 45 mg	Fiber: 2.1 g	Sodium: 231 mg

Yield: 8 servings

LOAF

1½ pounds 96% lean ground beef

1 medium yellow onion, finely chopped

¼ cup finely chopped green bell pepper

1½ teaspoons crushed fresh garlic

2 tablespoons minced fresh parsley, or 2 teaspoons dried

¾ cup oat bran or quick-cooking oats

¼ cup unsalted tomato sauce

3 egg whites

1½ teaspoons dried Italian seasoning

¼ teaspoon ground black pepper

½ teaspoon salt (optional)

TOPPING

¾ cup unsalted tomato sauce

1 teaspoon sugar

½ teaspoon dried Italian seasoning

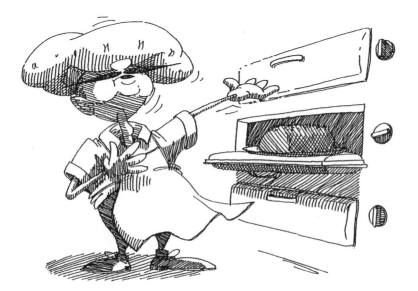

Choosing the Leanest Ground Meat

No food adds more fat to the diet than ground beef. And the wide range of choices now available—lean, extra-lean, ground round, ground sirloin, and ground chuck, for instance—does not seem to make it any easier to find a lean product. Complicating your choice is the fact that many package labels do not state fat content.

How fatty is ground beef? At its worst, ground beef is almost *33 percent pure fat.* Are ground chuck, sirloin, or round any leaner? Not necessarily. The terms chuck, sirloin, and round merely describe the part of the animal the meat is from; they do not indicate the amount of fat it contains. (Extra fat is often added during grinding.)

The only way to be sure about fat content is to buy meat in packages that provide some nutrition information. The leanest ground beef commonly available—96-percent lean ground beef—has only 1 gram of fat per ounce, and contains 4 percent fat by weight. Healthy Choice ground beef is an example. Most stores also carry ground beef that is 93-percent lean. This is also an acceptable choice. Another option is to select a lean piece of top round, and have the butcher trim off the visible fat and grind the remaining meat. Ground beef made this way is about 95-percent lean.

Where does ground turkey fit in? Ground turkey may be substituted for ground beef in any recipe—as long as you like the taste of ground turkey, which is distinctly different from that of beef. Realize, though, that ground turkey is not necessarily leaner than ground beef. In fact, much of the ground turkey sold today is 85 percent lean, meaning that it contains 15 percent fat by weight. This product contains *twice* the fat of 93-percent lean ground beef. How can ground turkey be so fatty? Often, this product contains turkey skin and fat, as well as turkey meat. So read the labels, and look for the lowest fat content available. Ground turkey made from dark meat without added skin or fat contains about 8 percent fat by weight. Ground turkey made from skinless breast meat contains only 1 percent fat. What about ground chicken?

Like ground turkey, it often contains added skin and fat, so, again, read the label before making your purchase.

The nutrition information for the ground beef recipes in this book has been calculated using Healthy Choice 96-percent lean ground beef. When you use ground meat this lean, there is no fat to drain off. In fact, the meat may stick to the bottom of the pan during browning. When this happens, add a few tablespoons of water to the skillet.

Using Meat Extenders and Substitutes

If your recipe allows you to drain the fat from your meat after browning—if you're making tacos or meat sauce, for instance—the degree of leaness is not that important, although fattier meats do shrink more during cooking. When making burgers or meat loaf, though, be sure to start with the leanest meat you can find. Then, if you like, reduce the fat even further by using one of two excellent beef extenders and substitutes.

The first product, texturized vegetable protein (TVP), is made from defatted soybean flour that is formed into small nuggets. You rehydrate TVP by mixing it with an equal amount of boiling water or broth. TVP is fat- and cholesterol-free, a good source of protein, and very economical. One ounce of hydrated TVP has only 26 calories and 0.1 grams of fat.

To mix TVP with ground meat, first combine a half cup of TVP with seven tablespoons of boiling water or broth. Let the mixture sit for about five minutes to hydrate, and then mix it with eight ounces of cooked ground meat to make one pound. When using TVP in spicy dishes like chili or tacos, you will not even know it's there. If you choose to use TVP in burgers or meat loaf, rehydrate the nuggets before mixing them with the uncooked beef. Then form the beef into patties or loaves, and cook as desired.

Another low-fat meat extender or substitute is Tofu Crumbles. These precooked, mildly seasoned, texturized bits can be found in the tofu section of most grocery stores. One ounce of Tofu Crumbles has 20 calories and 1.2 grams of fat. Ready to use, these crumbles can replace all or part of the ground beef in Sloppy Joes, tacos, spaghetti sauce, and chili. Simply add one cup of Tofu Crumbles to eight ounces of cooked ground meat to make one pound.

Fortunately, switching to a low-fat lifestyle does not mean giving up the foods you love. By choosing the lowest-fat products available, you can not only enjoy all of your favorite dishes, but also feel good about the foods you put on your table.

Saucy Stuffed Peppers

1. Place the meat in a large skillet, and cook over medium heat, stirring to crumble, until the meat is no longer pink. Stir in the onion, chili powder, pepper, and salt, if desired, and continue to cook and stir for a few more minutes, or until the onion is tender. (Add a few tablespoons of water or broth if the skillet gets too dry.) Remove the skillet from the heat, and stir in first the rice, and then the cheese.

2. Cut the tops off the peppers, and remove the seeds and membranes. Divide the filling among the peppers, and replace the pepper tops.

3. To make the sauce, combine all of the sauce ingredients in a large bowl, and stir to mix. Place the peppers upright in an 8-x-12-inch casserole dish or Dutch oven, and pour the sauce around the peppers. Cover with aluminum foil and bake at 350°F for 1 hour, or until the peppers are tender. Serve hot.

Yield: 8 servings

8 large green bell peppers

FILLING

1 pound 96% lean ground beef

1 medium onion, chopped

1 tablespoon chili powder

¼ teaspoon ground black pepper

½ teaspoon salt (optional)

4 cups cooked brown rice

1 cup shredded nonfat or reduced-fat Cheddar cheese

SAUCE

2 cans (1 pound each) unsalted tomato sauce

1 tablespoon chili powder

¼ teaspoon salt

NUTRITIONAL FACTS (PER SERVING)

Calories: 252	Fat: 3.2 g	Protein: 20 g
Cholesterol: 32 mg	Fiber: 4.8 g	Sodium: 334 mg

Mushroom and Onion Burgers

Yield: 6 servings

1 pound 96% lean ground beef

1½ cups chopped fresh mushrooms

½ cup chopped onion

1 cup soft whole wheat bread crumbs

2 tablespoons Worcestershire sauce

6 multigrain burger buns

TOPPINGS

6 slices tomato

6 thin slices onion

6 lettuce leaves

While these burgers cook, the chopped mushrooms and onions release their juices into the meat, keeping these ultra-lean burgers moist and flavorful.

1. Combine the ground beef, mushrooms, onions, bread crumbs, and Worcestershire sauce in a medium-sized bowl, and mix thoroughly. Gently shape the mixture into 6 (4-inch) patties.

2. Coat a large nonstick skillet with nonstick cooking spray, and preheat over medium heat. Place the patties in the skillet, and cook them for 4 to 5 minutes on each side, or until the meat is no longer pink inside. To cook the burgers on a barbecue grill, cook over medium heat for 7 to 9 minutes on each side, or until the meat is no longer pink inside.

3. Place each burger on a bun, and top with a slice of tomato, a slice of onion, and a lettuce leaf. Serve hot.

NUTRITIONAL FACTS (PER BURGER WITH BUN AND TOPPINGS)

Calories: 247	Fat: 4.1 g	Protein: 24 g
Cholesterol: 40 mg	Fiber: 4.8 g	Sodium: 521 mg

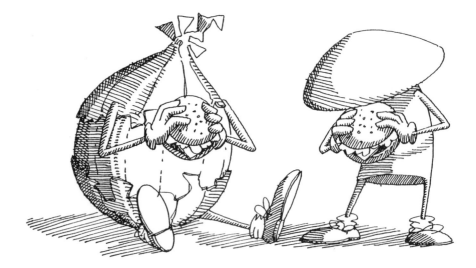

Shepherd's Pie

1. To make the topping, peel the potatoes and cut them into 1-inch pieces. Place in a 2-quart pot, barely cover with water, and bring to a boil over high heat. Reduce the heat to medium, cover, and cook for 10 minutes, or until the potatoes are soft.

2. Drain all but 2 tablespoons of water from the potatoes, reserving the drained water. Add the sour cream or yogurt, salt, and pepper, and mash the potatoes with a potato masher until smooth. If the potatoes are too stiff, add a little of the reserved cooking liquid. Set aside.

3. Place the meat in a large, deep skillet, and cook over medium heat, stirring to crumble, until the meat is no longer pink. Stir in the tomato sauce, chili powder, oregano, and bouillon granules, if desired, and continue to cook and stir just until the mixture is heated through.

4. Coat a $2\frac{1}{2}$-quart casserole dish with nonstick cooking spray, and spoon the beef mixture into the dish. Arrange the mixed vegetables in a layer over the beef mixture. Then spread the mashed potatoes over the vegetables. Top with the shredded cheese.

5. Bake uncovered at 350°F for 35 minutes, or until the edges are bubbly and the cheese is melted. Remove the dish from the oven, and let sit for 5 minutes before serving.

Yield: 6 servings

1 pound 96% lean ground beef

$1\frac{1}{2}$ cups unsalted tomato sauce

2 teaspoons chili powder

$\frac{1}{2}$ teaspoon dried oregano

1 teaspoon beef bouillon granules (optional)

1 package (10 ounces) frozen mixed vegetables, thawed

TOPPING

$1\frac{1}{2}$ pounds baking potatoes (about 4 medium)

$\frac{1}{2}$ cup nonfat sour cream or plain nonfat yogurt

$\frac{1}{4}$ teaspoon salt

$\frac{1}{8}$ teaspoon ground white pepper

1 cup shredded nonfat or reduced-fat Cheddar cheese

NUTRITIONAL FACTS (PER $1\frac{1}{3}$-CUP SERVING)		
Calories: 265	Fat: 3 g	Protein: 25 g
Cholesterol: 43 mg	Fiber: 5 g	Sodium: 451 mg

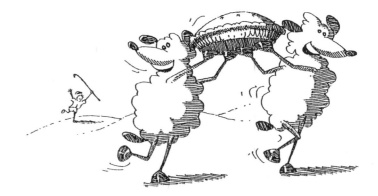

Sweet and Sour Pork

Yield: 5 servings

1-pound pork tenderloin

½ teaspoon crushed fresh garlic

1 can (20 ounces) pineapple chunks in juice, undrained

1 medium green bell pepper, cut into thin strips

1 medium yellow onion, cut into thin wedges

1 medium carrot, peeled and diagonally sliced

SAUCE

¼ cup chicken broth

¼ cup white wine vinegar or rice wine vinegar

2 tablespoons reduced-sodium soy sauce

2 tablespoons brown sugar

2 tablespoons cornstarch

½ teaspoon ground ginger

1. To make the sauce, combine all of the sauce ingredients in a small dish. Set aside.

2. Trim the tenderloin of any visible fat and membranes. Rinse with cool water, and pat dry with paper towels. Cut the tenderloin into 1-inch cubes, and set aside.

3. Coat a large nonstick skillet with nonstick cooking spray, and preheat over medium-high heat. Add the garlic and pork, and stir-fry for 5 to 6 minutes, or until the pork is browned.

4. Drain the juice from the pineapple, reserving both the juice and the fruit. Add the juice to the pork mixture, and bring to a boil. Reduce the heat to low, cover, and simmer for 6 to 8 minutes, or until the pork is tender and cooked through.

5. Add the pineapple chunks, bell pepper, onion, and carrot to the pork mixture. Cover and simmer for 3 additional minutes, or until the vegetables are crisp-tender.

6. Stir the sauce to mix, and add it to the skillet. Cook, stirring constantly, until the sauce is thickened and bubbly. Serve hot, accompanying the dish with brown rice, if desired.

NUTRITIONAL FACTS (PER 1-CUP SERVING)		
Calories: 226	Fat: 3.5 g	Protein: 20 g
Cholesterol: 54 mg	Fiber: 2 g	Sodium: 292 mg

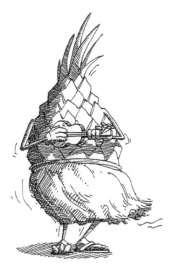

10. Meatless Main Dishes

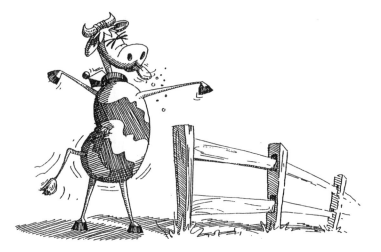

No one can dispute the health benefits of meatless eating. People who eat diets rich in veggies and low in meat have a reduced risk of heart disease, high blood pressure, obesity—the list goes on and on. And meatless dishes can be both delicious and satisfying. Pastas, whole grains, beans, low- and no-fat cheeses, garden-fresh vegetables, and herbs and spices can be combined to make dishes that are substantial enough for the largest of appetites, and flavorful enough for the fussiest of eaters.

Can you get all the protein you need without eating meat? Most definitely. Properly planned vegetarian meals that feature beans, grains, non-fat or low-fat dairy products, and egg whites or fat-free egg substitutes provide plenty of protein. In fact, one of the pitfalls of the typical American meat-based diet is that it provides *too much* protein, with many people eating almost twice the recommended amount. This level of protein can increase calcium loss from the body and contribute to osteoporosis, as well as causing a variety of other health problems. Most meats also provide far too much saturated fat and cholesterol—substances that should be sharply reduced in a healthy diet.

Of course, vegetarian meals made with full-fat cheeses, butter, oils, and egg yolks are no better than meals made with fatty meats. Fortunately, meatless meals can easily be made free of fat and cholesterol, and rich in fiber. The recipes in this chapter use nonfat dairy products, egg whites, and egg substitutes to reduce or totally eliminate the fat from a variety of dishes. The result? Rich and creamy quiches, golden macaroni and cheese, crusty pizza, and many other family favorites, all with no added fat. You'll be delighted to find that even luscious burgers and hearty chili can be made without meat. So if you're trying to eliminate meat from your diet—or if you simply want a change from the usual lunch and dinner fare—you've come to the right place. In the following pages, you'll find a variety of dishes that will prove to you once and for all that dishes made without meat can be not only healthful and low in fat, but also absolutely delicious.

Spring Vegetable Quiche
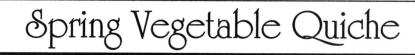

Yield: 5 servings

1½ cups cooked brown rice

1 egg white

1 cup chopped fresh asparagus or broccoli

½ cup fresh or frozen (thawed) whole kernel corn

⅓ cup finely chopped carrots

⅓ cup chopped fresh mushrooms

¼ cup finely chopped onion

2 tablespoons minced fresh parsley

1 cup shredded nonfat or reduced-fat mozzarella cheese

1 cup evaporated skim milk

1 cup fat-free egg substitute

2 tablespoons grated nonfat or reduced-fat Parmesan cheese

1. To make the crust, combine the brown rice and egg white in a medium-sized bowl, and stir to mix well. Coat a 9-inch deep dish pie pan with nonstick cooking spray, and use the back of a spoon to pat the mixture over the bottom and sides of the pan, forming an even crust.

2. Combine all of the remaining ingredients except for the Parmesan in a large bowl. Stir to mix well, and pour into the rice crust. Sprinkle the Parmesan over the top.

3. Bake at 375°F for about 50 minutes, or until the top is golden brown and a sharp knife inserted in the center of the quiche comes out clean. Remove the dish from the oven, and let sit for 5 minutes before slicing and serving.

NUTRITIONAL FACTS (PER SERVING)

Calories: 197	Fat: 0.9 g	Protein: 20 g
Cholesterol: 8 mg	Fiber: 2.5 g	Sodium: 337 mg

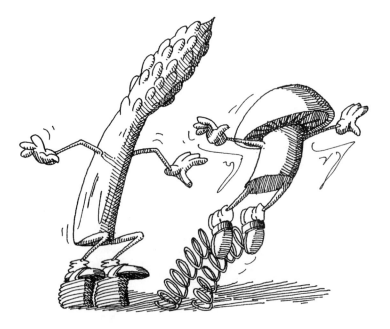

Spinach and Barley Bake

For variety, substitute brown rice or bulgur wheat for the barley.

Yield: 4 servings

1. Combine the barley and water in a 1½-quart pot, and bring to a boil over high heat. Reduce the heat to low, cover, and simmer for 45 to 50 minutes, or until the barley is tender and the liquid has been absorbed.

2. Combine the cooked barley and all of the remaining ingredients except for 2 tablespoons of the Parmesan in a large bowl, and stir to mix well. Coat a 1½-quart casserole dish with nonstick cooking spray, and spread the mixture evenly in the dish. Sprinkle the remaining Parmesan over the top.

3. Bake uncovered at 375°F for 50 to 60 minutes, or until golden brown and bubbly. Remove the dish from the oven, and let sit for 5 minutes before serving.

⅔ cup hulled barley

1⅔ cups water

1 package (10 ounces) frozen chopped spinach, thawed and squeezed dry

1 cup sliced fresh mushrooms

1 teaspoon crushed fresh garlic

1½ cups dry curd or nonfat cottage cheese

¼ cup plus 2 tablespooons grated nonfat or reduced-fat Parmesan cheese, divided

½ cup fat-free egg substitute

1 tablespoon unbleached flour

½ teaspoon dried thyme

⅛ teaspoon ground black pepper

NUTRITIONAL FACTS (PER 1¼-CUP SERVING)

Calories: 211	Fat: 0.8 g	Protein: 20 g
Cholesterol: 11 mg	Fiber: 5.9 g	Sodium: 188 mg

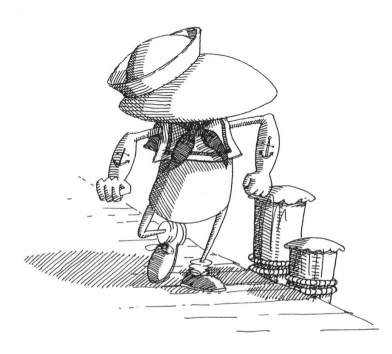

Baked Macaroni and Cheese

Yield: 6 servings

8 ounces elbow macaroni

2 cups skim milk, divided

2 tablespoons unbleached flour

$\frac{1}{4}$ teaspoon ground white pepper

2 teaspoons dry mustard

2 cups shredded nonfat processed Cheddar cheese, or 2 cups shredded reduced-fat Cheddar cheese, divided

1. Cook the macaroni al dente according to package directions. Drain, rinse, and drain again. Set aside.

2. Place $\frac{1}{2}$ cup of the milk and all of the flour, pepper, and mustard in a jar with a tight-fitting lid. Shake until smooth, and set aside.

3. Pour the remaining $1\frac{1}{2}$ cups of milk into a 2-quart pot, and bring to a boil over medium heat, stirring constantly. Add the flour mixture, and cook, still stirring, for about 1 minute, or until thickened and bubbly. Reduce the heat to low, add $1\frac{1}{2}$ cups of the cheese, and stir until the cheese melts.

4. Remove the pot from the heat, and stir in the macaroni. Coat a 2-quart casserole dish with nonstick cooking spray, and spread the macaroni mixture evenly in the dish. Sprinkle the remaining cheese over the top, and bake at 350°F for 30 to 35 minutes, or until bubbly around the edges. Remove the dish from the oven, and let sit for 5 minutes before serving.

NUTRITIONAL FACTS (PER 1-CUP SERVING)		
Calories: 232	Fat: 0.7 g	Protein: 20 g
Cholesterol: 8 mg	Fiber: 1 g	Sodium: 338 mg

FAT-FREE COOKING TIP

Cooking With Nonfat Cheeses

If you have been cooking with nonfat cheese for a while, you may have noticed that some brands do not melt as well as their full-fat counterparts. So how can you prepare a creamy nonfat cheese sauce, like the one in Baked Macaroni and Cheese? One option is to use a finely shredded brand of nonfat cheese. Finely shredded cheeses melt better than coarsely shredded products—although they still may not melt completely. Or use a processed nonfat cheese. Processed cheeses are specially made to melt, and will work in any sauce recipe. Processed cheeses tend to be higher in sodium than natural cheeses, though, so read labels and check the sodium counts before you make your purchase.

What about reduced-fat cheeses? Most brands melt very well and can be substituted for full-fat brands in any recipe, with very little difference in taste or texture. Only your waistline will know the difference!

Top: Eggplant Parmesan (page 138)
Center: Baked Macaroni and Cheese (page 136)
Bottom: Spring Vegetable Quiche (page 134)

Top: Bean Burritos Supreme (page 144)
Center: Two-Bean Chili (page 143)
Bottom: Fresh Tomato Pizza (page 139)

Top: Macaroon Swirl Cake (page 156)
Bottom Left: Chocolate Cherry Tunnel Cake (page 157)
Bottom Right: Blueberry Swirl Cheesecake (page 162)

Top: Razzleberry Trifle (page 167)
Bottom Left: Refreshing Fruit Pie (page 168)
Bottom Right: Pear Ginger Cake (page 159)

Fat-Free Eggs Foo Yung

For variety, make a nonvegetarian version by adding 1 cup of chopped cooked shrimp or crab meat.

1. To make the sauce, combine the cornstarch and brown sugar in a 1-quart saucepan, and stir to mix well. Add the broth, the soy or hoison sauce, and the sesame oil. Place the pan over medium heat, and cook, stirring constantly, until thickened and bubbly. Cover to keep warm, and set aside.

2. Combine the egg substitute, sprouts, water chestnuts, scallions, and pepper in a large bowl, and stir to mix well.

3. Coat a griddle or large skillet with nonstick cooking spray, and preheat over medium heat. For each pancake, pour $\frac{1}{2}$ cup of the egg mixture onto the griddle, spreading the bean sprouts out evenly to make a 4-inch cake. Cook for 3 minutes, or until the eggs are almost set. Flip the pancake over, and cook for 2 additional minutes, or until the eggs are completely set. As the pancakes are done, transfer them to a serving plate and keep warm in a preheated oven.

4. Serve hot, topping each serving with some of the sauce.

Yield: 4 servings

1$\frac{1}{2}$ cups fat-free egg substitute

4 cups mung bean sprouts

1 can (8 ounces) water chestnuts, drained and chopped

2 scallions, thinly sliced

$\frac{1}{8}$ teaspoon ground black pepper

SAUCE

2 teaspoons cornstarch

1 teaspoon brown sugar

1 cup unsalted vegetable broth

2 tablespoons reduced-sodium soy sauce or hoison sauce

$\frac{1}{2}$ teaspoon sesame oil

NUTRITIONAL FACTS (PER 2-PANCAKE SERVING)

Calories: 88	Fat: 0.6 g	Protein: 10 g
Cholesterol: 0 mg	Fiber: 1.3 g	Sodium: 411 mg

Eggplant Parmesan

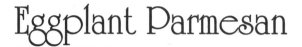

Yield: 6 servings

2 medium eggplants (about 1 pound each)

4 egg whites, beaten

½ cup dried Italian bread crumbs

¼ cup unbleached flour

½ cup grated nonfat or reduced-fat Parmesan cheese, divided

Olive oil cooking spray

1 cup shredded nonfat or reduced-fat mozzarella cheese

SAUCE

2 cans (1 pound each) unsalted tomatoes, crushed

1 can (6 ounces) tomato paste

1 medium onion, chopped

1½ teaspoons crushed fresh garlic

2 teaspoons dried Italian seasoning

¼ teaspoon ground black pepper

¼ teaspoon crushed red pepper

1. To make the sauce, combine all of the sauce ingredients in a 2-quart saucepan, and stir to mix well. Bring the mixture to a boil over high heat. Then reduce the heat to low, cover, and simmer for 20 minutes. Set aside to keep warm.

2. Trim the ends off the eggplants, but do not peel. Cut each eggplant crosswise into 9 slices, each approximately ½-inch thick.

3. Place the egg whites in a medium-sized shallow bowl. Combine the bread crumbs, flour, and ¼ cup of the Parmesan in another shallow bowl. Dip the eggplant slices first in the egg whites, and then in the crumb mixture.

4. Coat a large baking sheet with olive oil cooking spray, and arrange the eggplant slices in a single layer on the pan. Spray the tops of the slices very lightly with the cooking spray, and bake at 400°F for 15 to 20 minutes, or until the eggplant is golden brown and tender.

5. Coat a 9-x-13-inch baking pan with nonstick cooking spray. Transfer the eggplant slices to the dish, slightly overlapping the slices to allow them to fit in a single layer. Pour the sauce over the eggplant slices, and sprinkle with the mozzarella and the remaining Parmesan.

6. Bake at 400°F for 5 minutes, or until the cheese is melted. Serve hot with your choice of pasta.

NUTRITIONAL FACTS (PER SERVING)

Calories: 201	Fat: 1.1 g	Protein: 15 g
Cholesterol: 10 mg	Fiber: 6 g	Sodium: 588 mg

Time-Saving Tip

To reduce preparation time, make Eggplant Parmesan with 4½ cups of bottled fat-free marinara sauce instead of using homemade sauce.

Fresh Tomato Pizza

1. To make the crust, combine 1 cup of the flour with the oat bran, yeast, sugar, and salt, and stir to mix well. Place the water in a saucepan, and heat until very warm (125°F to 130°F). Add the water to the flour mixture, and stir for 1 minute. Stir in enough of the remaining flour, 2 tablespoons at a time, to form a stiff dough.

2. Sprinkle 2 tablespoons of the remaining flour over a flat surface, and turn the dough onto the surface. Knead the dough for 5 minutes, gradually adding enough of the remaining flour to form a smooth, satiny ball. Coat a large bowl with nonstick cooking spray, and place the dough in the bowl. Cover the bowl with a clean kitchen towel, and let rise in a warm place for about 35 minutes, or until doubled in size.

3. When the dough has risen, punch it down, shape it into a ball, and turn it onto a lightly floured surface. Using a rolling pin, roll the dough into a 12-inch circle. Sprinkle the cornmeal over a 12-inch pizza pan, and place the dough in the pan.

4. Spread the garlic over the crust. Then arrange a single layer of tomato slices over the garlic, extending the tomatoes to within $\frac{1}{2}$ inch of the edges. Sprinkle a layer of mozzarella over the tomatoes, and top with the pepper and onion rings. Finally, sprinkle with the oregano and Parmesan.

5. Bake at 450°F for 16 to 18 minutes, or until the cheese is browned and bubbly. Slice and serve immediately.

Yield: 8 slices

CRUST

1$\frac{3}{4}$ cups bread flour, divided

$\frac{1}{2}$ cup oat bran

1$\frac{1}{2}$ teaspoons Rapid Rise yeast

1 teaspoon sugar

$\frac{1}{4}$ teaspoon salt

$\frac{3}{4}$ cup water

1 teaspoon whole grain cornmeal

TOPPINGS

1 teaspoon crushed fresh garlic

3 large plum tomatoes, thinly sliced

1$\frac{1}{4}$ cups shredded nonfat or reduced-fat mozzarella cheese

8 thin green bell pepper rings

3 thin onion slices, separated into rings

1$\frac{1}{2}$ teaspoons dried oregano or Italian seasoning

1 tablespoon nonfat or reduced-fat Parmesan cheese

NUTRITIONAL FACTS (PER SLICE)		
Calories: 153	Fat: 0.8 g	Protein: 10 g
Cholesterol: 4 mg	Fiber: 2.3 g	Sodium: 189 mg

Time-Saving Tip

To make the dough for Fresh Tomato Pizza in a bread machine, place all of the dough ingredients in the machine's bread pan. (Do not heat the water.) Turn the machine to the "rise," "dough," or "manual" setting so that the machine will mix, knead, and let the dough rise once. Check the dough 5 minutes after the machine has started. If it seems too sticky, add more flour, a tablespoon at a time. If it seems too stiff, add more water. When the dough is ready, remove it from the machine and proceed to shape, top, and bake it as directed in the recipe.

Spinach and Cheese Calzones

Yield: 6 servings

CRUST

2¼ cups bread flour, divided

⅔ cup oat bran

1½ teaspoons Rapid Rise yeast

1 teaspoon sugar

¼ teaspoon salt

¼ teaspoon celery seed

1 cup water

1 teaspoon whole grain cornmeal

FILLING

1¼ cups chopped fresh spinach

2 tablespoons finely chopped onion

1¼ cups nonfat ricotta cheese

¾ cup grated nonfat or reduced-fat mozzarella cheese

2 tablespoons grated Parmesan cheese

¾ teaspoon dried Italian seasoning

SAUCE (OPTIONAL)

2 cups bottled fat-free marinara sauce

1. To make the crust, in a large bowl, combine 1¼ cups of the flour with all of the oat bran, yeast, sugar, salt, and celery seed, and stir to mix well. Place the water in a saucepan, and heat until very warm (125°F to 130°F). Add the water to the flour mixture, and stir for 1 minute. Stir in enough of the remaining flour, 2 tablespoons at a time, to form a stiff dough.

2. Sprinkle 2 tablespoons of the remaining flour over a flat surface, and turn the dough onto the surface. Knead the dough for 5 minutes, gradually adding enough of the remaining flour to form a smooth, satiny ball. Coat a large bowl with nonstick cooking spray, and place the dough in the bowl. Cover the bowl with a clean kitchen towel, and let rise in a warm place for about 35 minutes, or until doubled in size.

3. When the dough has risen, punch it down, divide it into 6 portions, and shape each portion into a ball. Using a rolling pin, roll each ball into a 7-inch circle.

4. To make the filling, combine all of the filling ingredients in a medium-sized bowl, and stir to mix well. Spread ⅙ of the filling on the bottom half of each circle of dough, extending the filling to within ½ inch of the edges. Brush a little water around the outer edges of each circle, fold the top half over the bottom half, and firmly press the edges together to seal.

5. Sprinkle the cornmeal over a large baking sheet, and arrange the calzones on the sheet. Bake at 450°F for 15 to 17 minutes, or until golden brown. If desired, place the marinara sauce in a small saucepan, and cook over medium heat just until heated through. Serve the calzones hot, accompanying each serving with a small dish of the warm sauce.

NUTRITIONAL FACTS (PER CALZONE)

Calories: 264	Fat: 1 g	Protein: 19.4 g
Cholesterol: 13 mg	Fiber: 3.5 g	Sodium: 336 mg

Time-Saving Tip:

Like the Fresh Tomato Pizza dough, the dough for Spinach and Cheese Calzones may be mixed in a bread machine. Just follow the directions on page 139.

Zucchini-Rice Casserole

1. Coat a large skillet with nonstick cooking spray, and add the zucchini, mushrooms, onions, tomatoes, and garlic. Place the skillet over medium heat, and cook, stirring constantly, for several minutes, or until the vegetables are tender and most of the liquid has evaporated.

2. Remove the skillet from the heat, and set aside to cool slightly. Stir in first the rice, and then the egg substitute, yogurt, Swiss or mozzarella, and pepper.

3. Coat a 2-quart casserole dish with nonstick cooking spray, and spread the mixture evenly in the dish. Sprinkle the Parmesan over the top, and bake at 350°F for about 50 minutes, or until browned and bubbly. Remove the dish from the oven, and let sit for 5 minutes before serving.

Yield: 6 servings

2 medium zucchini, scrubbed, halved lengthwise, and cut into $\frac{1}{4}$-inch slices

$1\frac{1}{2}$ cups sliced fresh mushrooms

$\frac{1}{2}$ cup chopped onion

2 medium plum tomatoes, chopped

1 teaspoon crushed fresh garlic

3 cups cooked brown rice

$\frac{1}{2}$ cup fat-free egg substitute

$\frac{1}{2}$ cup plain nonfat yogurt

1 cup shredded nonfat or reduced-fat Swiss or mozzarella cheese

$\frac{1}{4}$ teaspoon ground black pepper

3 tablespoons grated nonfat or reduced-fat Parmesan cheese

NUTRITIONAL FACTS (PER $1\frac{1}{4}$-CUP SERVING)		
Calories: 174	Fat: 1 g	Protein: 13 g
Cholesterol: 6 mg	Fiber: 3 g	Sodium: 199 mg

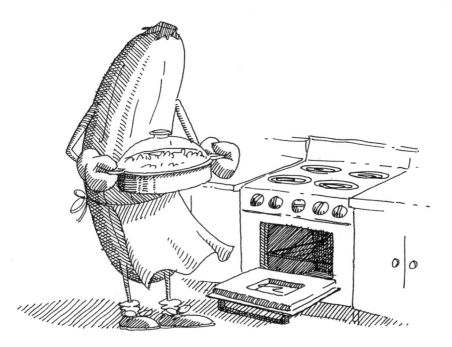

Broccoli Quiche in Potato Crust

Yield: 5 servings

1 package (10 ounces) frozen chopped broccoli, thawed and squeezed dry

1 cup shredded nonfat or reduced-fat Cheddar or Swiss cheese

1 cup dry curd or nonfat cottage cheese

1 cup fat-free egg substitute

¼ cup finely chopped onion

1½ teaspoons Dijon mustard

⅛ teaspoon ground black pepper

2 medium potatoes, scrubbed

1. Combine all of the ingredients except for the potatoes in a large bowl, and stir to mix well. Set aside.

2. Coat a 9-inch deep dish pie pan with nonstick cooking spray. Slice the potatoes ¼-inch thick, and arrange the slices in a single layer over the bottom and sides of the pan to form a crust. Pour the broccoli mixture into the crust.

3. Bake at 375°F for about 45 minutes, or until the top is golden brown and a sharp knife inserted in the center of the quiche comes out clean. Remove the dish from the oven, and let sit for 5 minutes before slicing and serving.

NUTRITIONAL FACTS (PER SERVING)

Calories: 175	Fat: 0.4 g	Protein: 20 g
Cholesterol: 6 mg	Fiber: 3.5 g	Sodium: 289 mg

Chili Cheese Casserole

Yield: 6 servings

5 cups cooked brown rice

6 fresh or canned (drained) mild green chili or banana peppers, diced into ¾-inch pieces

1¼ cups shredded nonfat or reduced-fat Monterey jack or Cheddar cheese

1½ teaspoons ground cumin

¼ teaspoon salt (optional)

1. Combine all of the ingredients in a large bowl, and stir to mix well.

2. Coat a 2-quart casserole dish with nonstick cooking spray, and spread the mixture evenly in the dish. Cover with aluminum foil, and bake at 350°F for 50 to 60 minutes, or until the peppers are tender and the dish is heated through. Serve hot.

NUTRITIONAL FACTS (PER 1-CUP SERVING)

Calories: 223	Fat: 1.4 g	Protein: 13 g
Cholesterol: 5 mg	Fiber: 3.1 g	Sodium: 208 mg

Two-Bean Chili

1. Combine the TVP and broth in a 3-quart pot, and bring to a boil over high heat. Remove the pot from the heat, and let sit for 5 minutes, or until the liquid has been absorbed.

2. Add all of the remaining ingredients except for the cheese to the TVP mixture, and stir to mix well. Place over high heat, and bring to a boil. Reduce the heat to low, cover, and simmer for 25 to 30 minutes, or until the vegetables are tender.

3. Serve hot, topping each serving with some of the cheese if desired.

Yield: 8 cups

1 cup texturized vegetable protein (TVP)

7/8 cup vegetable or beef broth

1 large onion, chopped

1 large green bell pepper, chopped

1 can (1 pound) unsalted tomatoes, crushed

1 can (1 pound) unsalted tomato sauce

1 can (1 pound) red kidney beans, drained

1 can (1 pound) pinto beans, drained

2–3 tablespoons chili powder

1 teaspoon dried oregano

1/2 teaspoon ground cumin

1 cup shredded nonfat or reduced-fat Cheddar cheese (optional)

NUTRITIONAL FACTS (PER 1-CUP SERVING)

Calories: 156	Fat: 0.8 g	Protein: 13 g
Cholesterol: 0 mg	Fiber: 11 g	Sodium: 302 mg

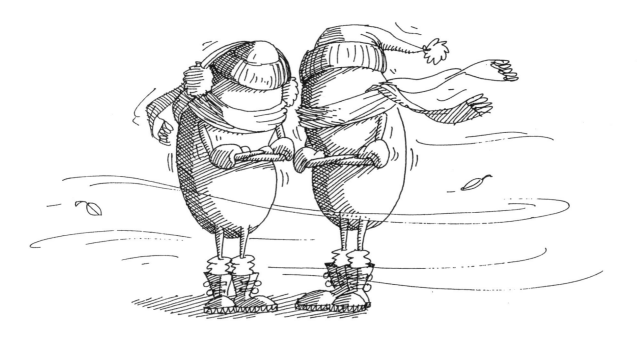

Bean Burritos Supreme

Yield: 6 servings

1¾ cups cooked pinto beans, or 1
   can (1 pound) pinto beans, drained

2 teaspoons chili powder

¼ teaspoon ground cumin

½ cup finely chopped yellow onion

½ cup finely chopped tomato

6 fat-free flour tortillas (10-inch
   rounds)

½ cup nonfat sour cream

½ cup shredded nonfat or
   reduced-fat Cheddar cheese

¾ cup shredded lettuce

NUTRITIONAL FACTS
(PER BURRITO)

Calories: 223	Fiber: 5.9 g
Chol: 2 mg	Protein: 10.2 g
Fat: 0.4 g	Sodium: 437 mg

---

1. Place the beans in a medium-sized bowl, and mash with a fork until slightly chunky. Stir in the chili powder and cumin, and set aside.

2. Coat a large skillet with nonstick cooking spray, and add the onion and tomato. Place the pan over medium heat, cover, and cook, stirring occasionally, for about 5 minutes, or until the vegetables are soft.

3. Add the beans to the skillet mixture, and cook uncovered, stirring constantly, until the beans are heated through and the mixture has the consistency of thick refried beans. Remove the skillet from the heat, cover to keep warm, and set aside.

4. Preheat a large nonstick skillet over medium-high heat, and place a tortilla in the skillet. To warm the tortilla, cook for 15 seconds, turning after 8 seconds.

5. Lay the warm tortilla on a flat surface, and spoon ¼ cup of the warm bean mixture along the right side of the tortilla. Top the bean mixture with 1 tablespoon of the sour cream, 1 tablespoon of the cheese, and 2 tablespoons of the lettuce. Fold the bottom edge of the tortilla up about 1 inch. (This fold will prevent the filling from falling out.) Then, beginning at the right edge, roll the tortilla up jelly-roll style.

6. Transfer the tortilla to a serving platter, cover with aluminum foil, and place in a 200°F oven to keep warm. Repeat with the remaining tortillas, and serve immediately.

**Making Bean Burritos
Supreme.**

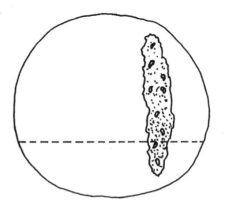

a. Arrange the filling along the
right side of the tortilla.

Black Bean Pizzas

1. Place the beans in a medium-sized bowl, and mash with a fork until slightly chunky. Stir in the chili powder, and set aside.

2. Coat a large skillet with nonstick cooking spray, and add the tomato and cumin. Place over medium heat, cover, and cook, stirring occasionally, for about 5 minutes, or until the tomatoes are soft.

3. Add the beans to the skillet, and cook uncovered, stirring constantly, until the beans are heated through and the mixture has the consistency of thick refried beans. Remove the skillet from the heat, and set aside.

4. Coat a large baking sheet with nonstick cooking spray, and lay the tortillas on the sheet. Spread $\frac{1}{4}$ cup of the bean mixture over each tortilla, extending the mixture to within $\frac{1}{2}$ inch of the edges. Top each tortilla with $\frac{1}{4}$ cup of the cheese, $\frac{1}{6}$ of the onions, $\frac{1}{6}$ of the olives, and 2 teaspoons of the jalapeños.

5. Bake uncovered at 400°F for 7 to 9 minutes, or until the pizzas are browned and crisp. Remove from the oven, top each pizza with 2 tablespoons each of the chopped tomato and shredded lettuce, and serve immediately.

Yield: 6 servings

1¾ cups cooked black beans, or 1 can (1 pound) black beans, drained

1 tablespoon chili powder

¾ cup finely chopped tomato

¼ teaspoon whole cumin seed

6 fat-free flour tortillas (10-inch rounds)

1½ cups shredded nonfat or reduced-fat Cheddar cheese

6 thin onion slices, separated into rings

6 large black olives, thinly sliced

2 tablespoons finely chopped jalapeño peppers (optional)

¾ cup chopped tomato

¾ cup shredded lettuce

NUTRITIONAL FACTS (PER PIZZA)		
Calories: 240	Fat: 1 g	Protein: 15.8 g
Cholesterol: 5 mg	Fiber: 6.2 g	Sodium: 585 mg

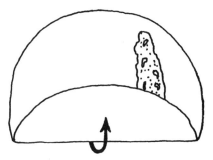

b. Fold the bottom edge of the tortilla up.

c. Fold the right side over the filling.

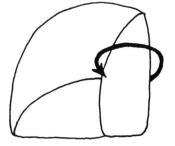

d. Continue folding to form a roll.

Lentil Chili

Yield: 8 cups

¾ cup dried brown lentils, cleaned (page 148)

2 cups chicken, beef, or vegetable broth

1 can (1 pound) unsalted tomatoes, crushed

1 medium green bell pepper, chopped

1 medium yellow onion, chopped

1 teaspoon crushed fresh garlic

2 tablespoons chili powder

½ teaspoon ground cumin

¼ teaspoon ground allspice

1 can (1 pound) unsalted tomato sauce

2 cups fresh or frozen (thawed) whole kernel corn

1. Combine all of the ingredients except for the tomato sauce and corn in a 2½-quart pot, and bring to a boil over high heat. Reduce the heat to low, cover, and simmer, stirring occasionally, for 25 to 30 minutes, or until the lentils are tender.

2. Add the tomato sauce and corn to the lentil mixture. Stir to mix, cover, and simmer for 10 to 15 additional minutes. Serve hot.

NUTRITIONAL FACTS (PER 1-CUP SERVING)

Calories: 140	Fat: 0.8 g	Protein: 9 g
Cholesterol: 0 mg	Fiber: 5.6 g	Sodium: 219 mg

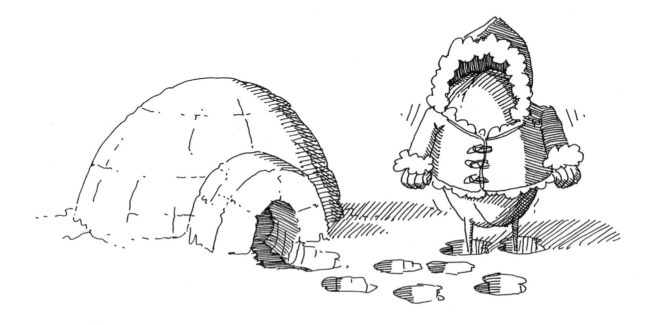

Bean Burgers

1. Combine the lentils, broth, and pepper in a 1½-quart pot, and bring to a boil over high heat. Reduce the heat to low, cover, and simmer for 25 to 30 minutes, or until the lentils are soft. Remove the pot from the heat, drain off any excess water, and set aside to cool.

2. While the lentils are cooking, tear the bread into pieces. Place the bread in a food processor or blender, and process into fine crumbs. Transfer the crumbs to a small dish, and set aside.

3. Place the cooked lentils in a food processor (this mixture is too stiff for a blender), and process until the mixture is almost smooth. Add the carrot, mushrooms, scallions, and bread crumbs, and process to mix well. Add the cheese, and process just until mixed.

4. Shape scant ½-cup portions of the lentil mixture into 6 (3½-inch) patties. Coat a large nonstick skillet or griddle with nonstick cooking spray, and preheat over medium heat. Place the patties in the skillet, and cook for 7 to 9 minutes, turning every 3 minutes, until golden brown.

5. Place each pattie in a pita pocket or bun, and top with 1 leaf of lettuce, 1 slice of tomato, 2 tablespoons of sprouts, and 1 tablespoon of ranch dressing. Serve immediately.

Yield: 6 servings

¾ cup dried brown lentils, cleaned (page 148)

1¾ cups unsalted vegetable or beef broth

¼ teaspoon ground black pepper

2 slices whole wheat bread

½ cup grated carrot

½ cup finely chopped fresh mushrooms

¼ cup finely chopped scallions

¾ cup shredded nonfat or reduced-fat Cheddar or mozzarella cheese

6 whole wheat pita pockets (6-inch rounds) or multigrain burger buns

6 lettuce leaves

6 slices tomato

¾ cup alfalfa sprouts

¼ cup plus 2 tablespoons bottled nonfat ranch dressing

NUTRITIONAL FACTS (PER BURGER)

Calories: 225	Fat: 1.6 g	Protein: 17 g
Cholesterol: 2 mg	Fiber: 7 g	Sodium: 440 mg

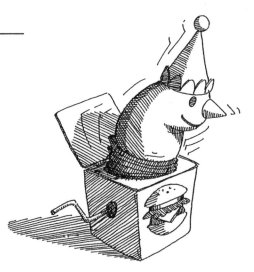

Bean Basics

If you really want to get the fat out of your diet, think beans. A hearty and satisfying alternative to meat, beans are fat-free, and rich in protein, complex carbohydrates, B vitamins, iron, zinc, copper, and potassium. As for fiber, no other food surpasses beans. Just a half cup of cooked beans provides 4 to 8 grams of fiber—up to four times the amount found in most other plant foods. Beans have also been found to lower cholesterol. As an added bonus, beans stabilize blood sugar levels, making you feel full and satisfied long after the meal is over—a definite benefit if you're watching your weight.

Some people avoid eating beans because of "bean bloat." What causes this problem? Complex sugars in beans, called oligosaccharides, sometimes form gas when broken down in the lower intestine. This side effect usually subsides when beans are made a regular part of the diet, and the body becomes more efficient at digesting them. The proper cleaning, soaking, and cooking of dried beans can also help prevent bean bloat. The following techniques will help you make beans a delicious and healthful part of your diet.

Cleaning

Because beans are a natural product, packages of dried beans sometimes contain shriveled or discolored beans, as well as small twigs and other items. Before cooking, sort through your beans and discard any discolored or blemished legumes. Rinse the beans well, cover them with water, and discard any that float to the top.

Soaking

There are two methods used to soak beans in preparation for cooking. If you have time—if you intend to cook your dish the next day, for instance—you may want to use the long method, as this technique is best for reducing the gas-producing oligosaccharides. If dinner is just a couple of hours away, though, the quick method is your best bet. Keep in mind that not all beans must be soaked before cooking. Black-eyed peas, brown and red lentils, and split peas do not require soaking.

The Long Method

After cleaning the beans, place them in a large bowl or pot, and cover them with four times as much water. Soak the beans for at least four hours, and for as long as twelve hours. If soaking them for more than four, place the bowl or pot in the refrigerator. After soaking, discard the water and replace with fresh water before cooking.

The Quick Method

After cleaning the beans, place them in a large pot, and cover them with four times as much water. Bring the pot to a boil over high heat, and continue to boil for two minutes. Remove the pot from the heat, cover, and let stand for one hour. After soaking, discard the water and replace with fresh water before cooking.

Cooking

To cook beans for use in salads, casseroles, and other dishes that contain little or no liquid, clean and soak as described above, discard the soaking water, and replace with two cups of water for each cup of dried beans. When beans are to be cooked in soups or stews that include acidic ingredients—lemon juice, vinegar, or tomatoes, for instance—add these ingredients at the end of the cooking time. Acidic foods can toughen the beans' outer layer, slowing the rate at which the beans cook. You'll know that the beans are done when you can mash them easily with a fork. Keep in mind that old beans may take longer to cook. During long cooking times, periodically check the pot, and add more liquid if necessary.

The following table gives approximate cooking times for several different beans. Need a meal in a hurry? Lentils and split peas require no soaking and cook quickly. Lentils are the fastest cooking of all the legumes; they can be ready in less than thirty minutes. Split peas cook in less than an hour.

Cooking Times for Dried Beans and Legumes

Bean or Legume	Cooking Time
Black, garbanzo, great northern, kidney, navy, pinto, and white beans	$1\frac{1}{2}$–2 hours
Black-eyed peas*	1–$1\frac{1}{4}$ hours
Lentils, brown*	25–30 minutes
Lentils, red*	15–20 minutes
Lima beans, baby	45 minutes–$1\frac{1}{4}$ hours
Lima beans, large	1–$1\frac{1}{2}$ hours
Split peas*	45–50 minutes

*These beans do not require soaking.

Curried Lentils

1. Place all of the ingredients in a $2\frac{1}{2}$-quart pot, and bring to a boil over high heat. Reduce the heat to low, cover, and simmer, stirring occasionally, for 25 to 30 minutes, or until the lentils are soft. (If you're using red lentils, cook the mixture for only 15 to 20 minutes.)

2. Serve hot, ladling each serving over brown rice or couscous, if desired.

Yield: 5 cups

1 cup dried brown or red lentils, cleaned (page 148)

3 cups unsalted chicken broth or water

1 large onion, chopped

2 medium carrots, peeled, halved, and sliced

2 stalks celery, thinly sliced (include leaves)

1 large apple, peeled and finely chopped

1 teaspoon crushed fresh garlic

$1\frac{1}{2}$ teaspoons chicken bouillon granules

2–3 teaspoons curry powder

NUTRITIONAL FACTS (PER 1-CUP SERVING)		
Calories: 181	Fat: 0.7 g	Protein: 12 g
Cholesterol: 0 mg	Fiber: 7.2 g	Sodium: 340 mg

Southwestern Black Beans

Yield: 8 servings

2½ cups black beans, cleaned and soaked (page 148)

7½ cups unsalted chicken broth or water

2 medium yellow onions, chopped

1 large green bell pepper, chopped

2 teaspoons crushed fresh garlic

2 teaspoons ham, chicken, or vegetable bouillon granules, or 6 ounces ham (at least 97% lean), diced

1 tablespoon chili powder

2 dried hot red chili pepper pods

1 teaspoon dried oregano

½ teaspoon ground cumin

¼ teaspoon ground black pepper

¼ cup distilled white vinegar

TOPPINGS

¾ cup shredded nonfat or reduced-fat Cheddar cheese

½ cup nonfat sour cream

¼ cup sliced scallions

1. Combine all of the ingredients except for the vinegar and toppings in a 4-quart pot, and bring to a boil over high heat. Reduce the heat to low, cover, and simmer, stirring occasionally, for 2 hours, or until the beans are soft and the liquid is thick. Periodically check the pot during cooking, and add a little more broth or water if needed.

2. Remove the pot from the heat, discard the pepper pods, and stir in the vinegar. Serve hot, topping each serving with a 1½ tablespoons of cheese, 1 tablespoon of sour cream, and 1½ teaspoons of scallions. If desired, serve over brown rice.

NUTRITIONAL FACTS (PER 1-CUP SERVING)		
Calories: 237	Fat: 0.8 g	Protein: 16 g
Cholesterol: 2 mg	Fiber: 16 g	Sodium: 345 mg

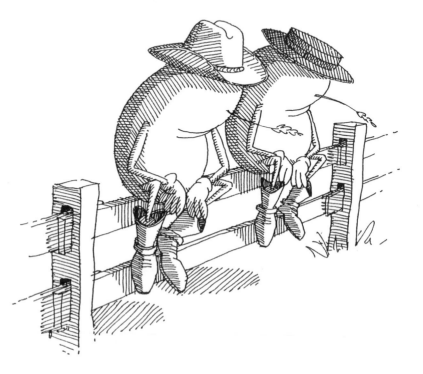

Spicy Pinto Beans

1. Combine all of the ingredients except for the tomatoes and cilantro in a 3-quart pot, and bring to a boil over high heat. Reduce the heat to low, cover, and simmer, stirring occasionally, for 1 hour and 30 minutes, or until the beans are tender. Periodically check the pot during cooking, and add a little more broth or water if needed.

2. Add the tomatoes to the bean mixture, and cook for 30 additional minutes. Serve hot, topping the beans with cilantro or scallions. If desired, serve over brown rice.

Yield: 7 cups

2 cups dried pinto beans, cleaned and soaked (page 148)

5½ cups unsalted chicken broth or water

1 medium onion, chopped

1 teaspoon crushed fresh garlic

1 tablespoon chopped jalapeño peppers

2 teaspoons ham, chicken, or vegetable bouillon granules

1½ teaspoons ground cumin

2 teaspoons chili powder

2 medium tomatoes, diced

⅓ cup chopped fresh cilantro or scallions

NUTRITIONAL FACTS (PER 1-CUP SERVING)

Calories: 184	Fat: 0.9 g	Protein: 11 g
Cholesterol: 0 mg	Fiber: 15 g	Sodium: 289 mg

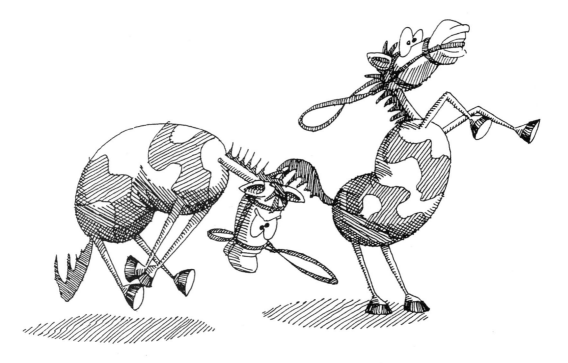

Jamaican Red Beans

Yield: 7 cups

2 cups dried red kidney beans,
 cleaned and soaked (page 148)

6 cups unsalted chicken broth or water

2 medium onions, chopped

2 stalks celery, thinly sliced (include
 leaves)

2 teaspoons ham or chicken bouillon
 granules

2 teaspoons dried thyme

½ teaspoon ground allspice

¼ teaspoon ground black pepper

2 bay leaves

2–3 dried hot red chili pepper pods

2 tablespoons distilled white vinegar

1. Combine all of the ingredients except for the vinegar in a 3-quart pot, and bring to a boil over high heat. Reduce the heat to low, cover, and simmer, stirring occasionally, for 2 hours, or until the beans are soft and the liquid is thick. Add a little more liquid during cooking if needed.

2. Remove the pot from the heat, and discard the bay leaves and pepper pods. Stir in the vinegar, and serve hot, ladling the beans over brown rice if desired.

NUTRITIONAL FACTS (PER 1-CUP SERVING)

Calories: 193	Fat: 0.6 g	Protein: 12 g
Cholesterol: 0 mg	Fiber: 12 g	Sodium: 247 mg

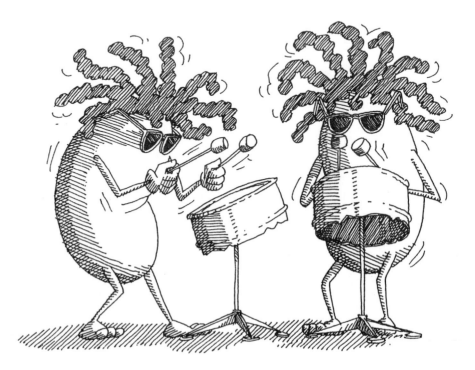

11. Sweet Stuff

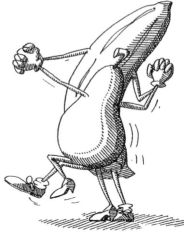

Everyone knows that desserts are full of sugar, but few people realize that the biggest danger desserts pose to our health—and our weight!—is their fat content. Fat generally contributes far more calories to desserts than sugar does. Consider the ingredients that might be used to make a chocolate cake, for instance. A cake whose batter includes 1 cup of sugar will get 770 calories and no fat from the sugar. Stir in 1 cup of oil, though, and you've added almost 2,000 calories, plus *224 grams of fat*! Of course, ingredients like egg yolks, cream cheese, heavy cream, and baking chocolate add even more fat and calories. And these are just a few of the ingredients considered essential for making great desserts.

The recipes in this chapter prove that all this fat simply is not necessary. In fact, most of these recipes contain no butter, margarine, or oil at all! Fruit purées, nonfat buttermilk and yogurt, liquid sweeteners like molasses, and other ingredients replace the fats traditionally used in baking—and do so with moist and flavorful results.

One of the pitfalls of many commerical fat-free desserts is that when fat is removed, extra sugar is added. In fact, many of the fat-free cookies, cakes, and other dessert items available today contain just as many calories as their high-fat counterparts do. The recipes in this book do not substitute sugar for fat. They do contain sugar, but the amount is 25 to 50 percent lower than that used in traditional recipes. Fruits and fruit juices; flavorings like vanilla extract, nutmeg, and cinnamon; and mildly sweet flours like oat flour have been used to reduce the need for sugar, and to add fiber and other nutrients, as well.

Of course, even though a dessert may be bursting with vitamins, minerals, and fiber, if it does not taste good, no one will eat it. You'll be delighted to discover that the low- and no-fat treats presented in this chapter are truly great-tasting. They are so moist and luscious, in fact, that no one but you will guess just how wholesome they are.

Before taking out your baking pans and preheating your oven, you might wish to turn to "About the Ingredients," on page 5. That section will acquaint you with the whole grain flours you'll be using, and will guide you in substituting less-refined sweeteners for traditional sweeteners, if you wish to do so. Then get ready to treat family and friends to bubbling fruit cobblers, creamy cheesecakes, moist and chewy fudge brownies, and more—all made absolutely delicious with the secrets of fat-free cooking.

Carrot-Pineapple Cake

Yield: 16 servings

2½ cups unbleached flour

1⅓ cups sugar

2 teaspoons baking soda

2 teaspoons ground cinnamon

2 cans (8 ounces each) crushed
   pineapple in juice, undrained

¼ cup skim milk

4 egg whites, lightly beaten, or ½ cup
   fat-free egg substitute

2 teaspoons vanilla extract

2 cups (packed) grated carrots (about
   5 medium)

½ cup golden raisins

⅓ cup chopped pecans (optional)

CREAM CHEESE ICING

8 ounces nonfat or reduced-fat cream
   cheese

1 cup nonfat ricotta cheese

½ cup confectioner's sugar

1 teaspoon vanilla extract

1. Combine the flour, sugar, baking soda, and cinnamon in a medium-sized bowl, and stir to mix well. Stir in the pineapple, including the juice, and the milk, egg whites, and vanilla extract. Fold in the carrots, raisins, and, if desired, the pecans.

2. Coat a 9-x-13-inch pan with nonstick cooking spray. Spread the batter evenly in the pan, and bake at 325°F for 35 minutes, or just until a wooden toothpick inserted in the center of the cake comes out clean. Cool to room temperature.

3. To make the icing, combine all of the icing ingredients in a food processor, and process until smooth. Spread the icing over the cake, and serve immediately. Refrigerate any leftovers.

NUTRITIONAL FACTS (PER SERVING)		
Calories: 215	Fat: 0.3 g	Protein: 7.7 g
Cholesterol: 3 mg	Fiber: 1.4 g	Sodium: 268 mg

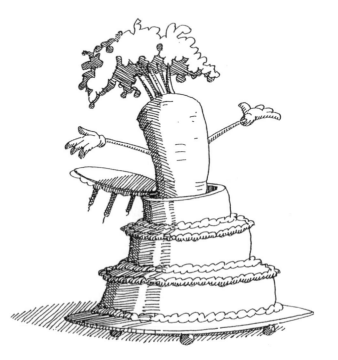

Minty Mocha-Fudge Cake

Yield: 16 servings

1. Combine the flours, sugar, cocoa, and baking soda in a large bowl, and stir to mix well. Set aside.

2. Combine the coffee, chocolate syrup, vinegar, and vanilla extract in a medium-sized bowl, and stir to mix well. Add the coffee mixture to the flour mixture, and stir with a wire whisk until well mixed.

3. Coat a 9-x-13-inch pan with nonstick cooking spray. Pour the batter into the pan, and bake at 350°F for 30 minutes, or just until a wooden toothpick inserted in the center of the cake comes out clean. Cool to room temperature.

4. To make the glaze, combine all of the glaze ingredients in a small bowl, and stir to mix well. If using a microwave oven, microwave the glaze, uncovered, at high power for 20 seconds, or until runny. If using a conventional stove top, combine the glaze ingredients in a small saucepan, and cook over medium heat, stirring constantly, for 20 seconds. Drizzle the glaze over the cake, and let the cake stand for at least 15 minutes, allowing the glaze to harden, before slicing and serving.

2 cups unbleached flour

1 cup oat flour

1½ cups sugar

½ cup cocoa powder

2 teaspoons baking soda

2 cups coffee, cooled to room temperature

½ cup chocolate syrup

1 tablespoon distilled white vinegar

2 teaspoons vanilla extract

GLAZE

1 cup confectioner's sugar

1 tablespoon cocoa powder

4 drops peppermint extract

4–5 teaspoons skim milk

NUTRITIONAL FACTS (PER SERVING)

Calories: 207	Fat: 1 g	Protein: 3.4 g
Cholesterol: 0 mg	Fiber: 2.4 g	Sodium: 168 mg

LOW-FAT COOKING TIP

Chocolate Flavor
With a Fraction of the Fat

For rich chocolate flavor with minimal fat, substitute cocoa powder for high-fat baking chocolate. Simply use three tablespoons of cocoa powder plus two teaspoons of water or another liquid to replace each ounce of baking chocolate in cakes, brownies, puddings, and other goodies. You'll save 111 calories and 13.5 grams of fat for each ounce of baking chocolate you replace!

Here's another fat-cutting tip for chocolate lovers. Replace the butter, margarine, or other solid shortening in chocolate cookies, cakes, brownies, and other baked goods with Prune Butter (page 160). Dark, sweet, nutritious, and fat-free, Prune Butter adds moistness and enhances the flavor of chocolate. You will never miss the fat!

Macaroon Swirl Cake

Yield: 16 servings

1/4 cup plus 2 tablespoons reduced-fat margarine or light butter

1 1/2 cups sugar

2 egg whites

1 1/2 teaspoons vanilla extract

2 cups unbleached flour

3/4 cup oat bran

1 1/4 teaspoons baking soda

1 1/4 cups plus 2 tablespoons nonfat buttermilk

1/4 cup sweetened flaked coconut

3/4 teaspoon coconut extract

1/4 cup plus 2 tablespoons cocoa powder

GLAZE

1/4 cup plus 2 tablespoons confectioner's sugar

1/2 teaspoon coconut extract

1 1/2 teaspoons skim milk

1 tablespoon sweetened flaked coconut

1. Place the margarine or butter and the sugar in the bowl of an electric mixer, and beat until smooth. Beat in the egg whites and vanilla extract until smooth, and set aside.

2. Combine the flour, oat bran, and baking soda in a medium-sized bowl, and stir to mix well. Add the flour mixture and the buttermilk to the margarine mixture, and beat just until well mixed.

3. Remove 1 cup of the batter, and place it in a small bowl. Stir in the flaked coconut and coconut extract, and set aside.

4. Add the cocoa to the large bowl of batter, and beat just until well mixed.

5. Coat a 12-cup bundt pan with nonstick cooking spray. Pour 3/4 of the cocoa batter into the pan, spreading the batter evenly. Top with the coconut batter, followed by the remaining cocoa batter.

6. Bake at 350°F for 40 minutes, or just until a wooden toothpick inserted in the center of the cake comes out clean. Cool the cake in the pan for 20 minutes. Then invert onto a wire rack, and cool to room temperature.

7. To make the glaze, combine the confectioner's sugar, coconut extract, and milk in a small bowl, and stir until smooth. Transfer the cake to a serving platter, and drizzle the glaze over the cake. Sprinkle the coconut over the top of the glaze, and let sit for at least 15 minutes, allowing the glaze to harden, before slicing and serving.

NUTRITIONAL FACTS (PER SERVING)

Calories: 189	Fat: 3.3 g	Protein: 4.1 g
Cholesterol: 0 mg	Fiber: 1.9 g	Sodium: 155 mg

Chocolate Cherry Tunnel Cake

1. Combine the flour, oat bran, sugar, cocoa, baking soda, and salt in a large bowl, and stir to mix well. Add the buttermilk, oil, egg whites, and vanilla extract, and stir to mix well.

2. Coat a 12-cup bundt pan with nonstick cooking spray, and spread the batter evenly in the pan. Spoon the cherry filling in a ring over the center of the batter. (As the cake bakes, the filling will sink into the batter.)

3. Bake at 350°F for about 40 minutes, or until the top springs back when lightly touched, and a wooden toothpick inserted near the sides of the cake comes out clean. Cool the cake in the pan for 40 minutes. Then invert onto a wire rack, and cool to room temperature.

4. To make the glaze, combine the confectioner's sugar, milk, and almond extract in a small bowl, and stir until smooth. Transfer the cake to a serving platter, and spoon the glaze over the cake. Let the cake sit for at least 15 minutes, allowing the glaze to harden, before slicing and serving.

Yield: 16 servings

1¾ cups unbleached flour

¾ cup oat bran

1⅓ cups sugar

½ cup cocoa powder

1½ teaspoons baking soda

⅛ teaspoon salt

1¼ cups nonfat buttermilk

3 tablespoons vegetable oil

2 egg whites, lightly beaten

1 teaspoon vanilla extract

FILLING

1¼ cups canned light (low-sugar) cherry pie filling

GLAZE

⅓ cup confectioner's sugar

1½ teaspoons skim milk

½ teaspoon almond extract

NUTRITIONAL FACTS (PER SERVING)

Calories: 188	Fat: 3.3 g	Protein: 4 g
Cholesterol: 0 mg	Fiber: 2.1 g	Sodium: 164 mg

LOW-FAT COOKING TIP

Slashing Fat in Half

To halve the fat in your baked goods, replace the butter, margarine, or other solid shortening in cakes, muffins, quick breads, cookies, and other treats with half as much oil. Bake as usual, checking the product for doneness a few minutes before the end of the usual baking time. This technique makes it possible to produce moist and tender cakes, breads, and biscuits; crisp cookies; and tender pie crusts—all with half the original fat.

Sour Cream Apple Coffee Cake

Yield: 8 servings

1 cup unbleached flour

½ cup whole wheat flour

½ cup sugar

1 teaspoon baking soda

½ teaspoon ground cinnamon

½ cup apple juice

¼ cup nonfat sour cream

1 egg white, lightly beaten

2½ cups thinly sliced peeled apples (about 3 medium)

¼ cup plus 2 tablespoons dark raisins

TOPPING

2 tablespoons light brown sugar

2 tablespoons toasted wheat germ or finely chopped walnuts

For variety, substitute sliced peaches or pears for the apples.

1. To make the topping, combine the brown sugar and wheat germ or nuts in a small bowl, and stir to mix well. Set aside.

2. Combine the flours, sugar, baking soda, and cinnamon in a medium-sized bowl, and stir to mix well. Stir in the apple juice, sour cream, and egg white. Fold in the apples and raisins.

3. Coat a 9-inch round pan with nonstick cooking spray, and spread the batter evenly in the pan. Sprinkle the topping over the batter, and bake at 350°F for 30 to 33 minutes, or just until a wooden toothpick inserted in the center of the cake comes out clean.

4. Cool the cake to room temperature, cut into wedges, and serve.

NUTRITIONAL FACTS (PER SERVING)

Calories: 163	Fat: 0.7 g	Protein: 4 g
Cholesterol: 0 mg	Fiber: 3.4 g	Sodium: 199 mg

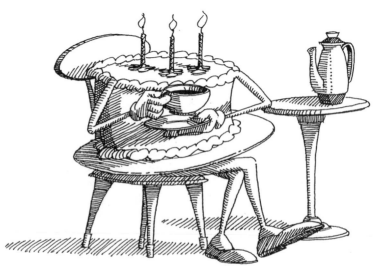

Pear Ginger Cake

For variety, substitute apricots or peaches for the pears.

Yield: 10 servings

1. Drain the pears, reserving the juice. Coat a 10-inch ovenproof skillet with nonstick cooking spray. Place $1\frac{1}{2}$ tablespoons of the reserved pear juice in the bottom of the skillet, and distribute evenly. Sprinkle the brown sugar evenly over the pear juice. Arrange 10 pear halves over the brown sugar, with the cut side down and the widest part of the pears pointing toward the outer edge of the skillet. Fill the center with walnut halves, if desired. Set aside.

2. Combine the flours, sugar, baking powder, baking soda, and spices in a medium-sized bowl, and stir to mix well. Combine the molasses, Prune Butter, and $\frac{3}{4}$ cup of the reserved pear juice in a medium-sized bowl, and stir to mix well. Add the molasses mixture and egg substitute to the flour mixture, and stir to mix well.

3. Bake at 350°F for 30 minutes, or just until a wooden toothpick inserted in the center of the cake comes out clean. Cool the cake in the skillet for 15 minutes. Then invert onto a serving platter. Cool to room temperature before slicing and serving.

2 cans (1 pound each) pear halves in juice, undrained

$\frac{1}{3}$ cup brown sugar

10 walnut halves (optional)

1 cup unbleached flour

$\frac{1}{2}$ cup whole wheat flour

$\frac{1}{4}$ cup sugar

1 teaspoon baking powder

$\frac{3}{4}$ teaspoon baking soda

$\frac{3}{4}$ teaspoon ground ginger

$\frac{1}{2}$ teaspoon ground cinnamon

$\frac{1}{4}$ teaspoon ground nutmeg

$\frac{1}{4}$ cup plus 2 tablespoons molasses

$\frac{1}{4}$ cup Prune Butter (page 160)

3 tablespoons fat-free egg substitute

NUTRITIONAL FACTS (PER SERVING)

Calories: 177	Fat: 0.3 g	Protein: 2.8 g
Cholesterol: 0 mg	Fiber: 2.2 g	Sodium: 147 mg

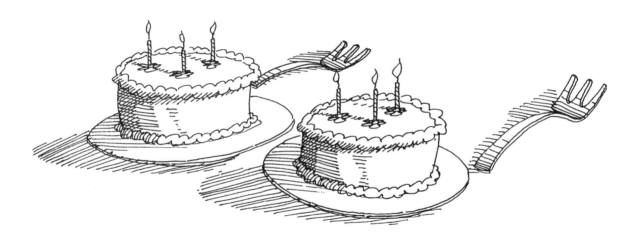

Making Prune Purée and Prune Butter

The dessert recipes in this book use a variety of substitutes, most of which are readily available in grocery stores. Two excellent fat substitutes, however, must be made at home. Prune Purée and Prune Butter will allow you to bake moist and flavorful cakes, cookies, and other treats with little or no fat, and will also add fiber and nutrients to your homemade goodies. Simply follow the recipes provided below, and keep these ingredients on hand for use in your fat-free baked goods.

Prune Purée

Yield: 1½ cups

3 ounces pitted prunes (about ½ cup)

1 cup water or fruit juice

2 teaspoons lecithin granules*

1. Place all of the ingredients in a blender or food processor, and process at high speed until the mixture is smooth.

2. Use immediately, or place in an airtight container and store in the refrigerator for up to 3 weeks.

Prune Butter

Yield: 1 cup

8 ounces pitted prunes (about 1⅓ cups)

6 tablespoons water or fruit juice

1. Place both ingredients in a food processor, and process at high speed until the mixture forms a smooth paste. (Note that this mixture is too thick to be made in a blender.)

2. Use immediately, or place in an airtight container and store in the refrigerator for up to 3 weeks.

*Lecithin, a nutritious by-product of soybean-oil refining, is sold in health foods stores as a food supplement. Because lecithin improves the texture of baked goods, commercial bakers often add small amounts of this product to fat-free and low-fat cakes, cookies, breads, and muffins.

Old-Fashioned Peach Cobbler

1. To make the filling, place the orange juice, sugar, cornstarch, cinnamon, and nutmeg in a 2-quart pot, and stir to mix well. Place the pot over medium heat, and cook, stirring constantly, for 3 to 5 minutes, or until the mixture is thickened and bubbly.

2. Remove the pot from the heat, and stir the peach slices into the glaze, tossing gently to coat. Coat a 2-quart casserole dish with nonstick cooking spray, and spread the peach mixture evenly in the dish.

3. To make the batter, place the flour, oat bran, sugar, baking powder, and baking soda in a medium-sized bowl, and stir to mix well. Stir in the buttermilk.

4. Spread the batter evenly over the fruit, and bake at 350°F for 35 to 40 minutes, or until the topping is golden brown and the filling is bubbly around the edges. (Loosely cover the dish with aluminum foil during the last 10 minutes of baking if the top starts to brown too quickly.) Remove the dish from the oven, and let stand for at least 10 minutes. Serve warm or at room temperature.

Yield: 8 servings

FRUIT FILLING

½ cup orange juice

¼ cup sugar

2 tablespoons cornstarch

¼ teaspoon ground cinnamon

⅛ teaspoon ground nutmeg

4½ cups sliced peeled peaches (about 5 medium), or 4½ cups frozen (thawed) sliced peaches

BATTER

¾ cup unbleached flour

⅓ cup oat bran

⅓ cup sugar

1½ teaspoons baking powder

½ teaspoon baking soda

¾ cup nonfat buttermilk

NUTRITIONAL FACTS (PER ¾-CUP SERVING)

Calories: 172	Fat: 0.6 g	Protein: 3.3 g
Cholesterol: 0 mg	Fiber: 2.7 g	Sodium: 172 mg

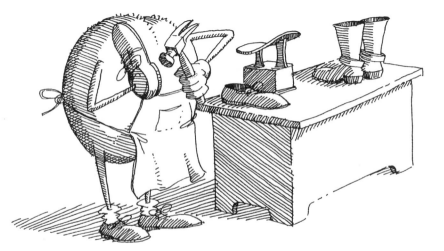

Cool and Creamy Cheesecake

Yield: 10 servings

CRUST

4½ large (2½-x-5-inch) fat-free or
reduced-fat graham crackers

1 tablespoon sugar

1 tablespoon fat-free egg substitute

FILLING

1 pound nonfat cream cheese,
softened to room temperature

15 ounces nonfat ricotta cheese

½ cup fat-free egg substitute

¾ cup sugar

¼ cup plus 2 tablespoons unbleached
flour

1 tablespoon freshly grated lemon
rind, or 1 teaspoon dried

2 teaspoons vanilla extract

NUTRITIONAL FACTS ➤
(PER SERVING)

Calories: 192	Fiber: 0.4 g
Chol: 10 mg	Protein: 14 g
Fat: 0.3 g	Sodium: 346 mg

NUTRITIONAL FACTS ➤
(PER SERVING)

Calories: 208	Fiber: 0.6 g
Chol: 10 mg	Protein: 14 g
Fat: 0.3 g	Sodium: 346 mg

---

1. To make the crust, break the crackers into pieces, and place in the bowl of a food processor or blender. Process into fine crumbs. Measure the crumbs. There should be ¾ cup. (Adjust the amount if necessary.)

2. Return the crumbs to the food processor or blender, add the sugar, and process for a few seconds to mix. Add the egg substitute, and process until the mixture is moist and crumbly.

3. Coat a 9-inch springform pan with nonstick cooking spray, and use the back of a spoon to press the mixture over the bottom of the pan and ½-inch up the sides, forming an even crust. (Periodically dip the spoon in sugar, if necessary, to prevent sticking.) Bake at 350°F for 8 minutes, or until the edges feel firm and dry. Set aside to cool.

4. To make the filling, place the cream cheese, ricotta, egg substitute, sugar, flour, lemon rind, and vanilla extract in a food processor, and process until smooth. Spread the filling evenly over the crust, and bake at 325°F for 1 hour, or until the center is set. Turn the oven off, and allow the cake to cool in the oven with the door ajar for 30 minutes.

5. Remove the cake from the oven, and chill for at least 8 hours. Remove the collar of the pan just before slicing and serving. Top each serving with fresh fruit or canned cherry pie filling if desired.

Variation

To make Blueberry Swirl Cheesecake, prepare the cheesecake crust and filling as directed above. Spread half of the cheesecake batter evenly over the crust. Then spoon ¾ cup of canned blueberry pie filling randomly over the batter. Top with the remaining batter, and draw a knife through the batter to produce a marbled effect. Bake as directed.

Pear-Raisin Crisp

1. To make the filling, combine the pear slices and raisins in a large bowl, and toss to mix well. Coat a 9-inch deep dish pie pan with nonstick cooking spray, and spread the fruit evenly in the pan. Set aside.

2. To make the topping, combine the cereal or walnuts, brown sugar, flour, cinnamon, and nutmeg in a medium-sized bowl, and stir to mix well. Add the juice concentrate, and stir until the mixture is moist and crumbly.

3. Sprinkle the topping over the fruit, and bake uncovered at 350°F for 50 minutes, or until the topping is browned and the filling is bubbly around the edges. Remove the dish from the oven, and let stand for at least 5 minutes. Serve warm or at room temperature.

Yield: 6 servings

FRUIT FILLING

5 cups sliced peeled pears (about 5 medium)

⅓ cup dark raisins

TOPPING

¼ cup barley nugget cereal or chopped walnuts

¼ cup light brown sugar

3 tablespoons whole wheat flour

⅛ teaspoon ground cinnamon

⅛ teaspoon ground nutmeg

1 tablespoon frozen apple juice concentrate, thawed

NUTRITIONAL FACTS (PER ¾-CUP SERVING)

Calories: 165	Fat: 0.6 g	Protein: 1.9 g
Cholesterol: 0 mg	Fiber: 4.5 g	Sodium: 36 mg

LOW-FAT COOKING TIP

Baking With Reduced-Fat Margarine and Light Butter

Contrary to popular belief, you *can* bake with reduced-fat margarine and light butter. These products make it possible to reduce fat by more than half and still enjoy light, tender, buttery-tasting cakes; crisp cookies; flaky pie crusts; and other goodies that are not easily made fat-free.

Because reduced-fat margarine and butter are diluted with water, they cannot be substituted for their full-fat counterparts on a one-for-one basis. To compensate for the extra water, substitute three-fourths as much of the light product for the full-fat butter or margarine. For instance, if the cake recipe calls for one cup of butter, use three-fourths cup of light butter. Be sure to choose a brand that contains 5 to 6 grams of fat and 50 calories per tablespoon. (Full-fat brands contain 11 grams of fat and 100 calories per tablespoon.) Brands with less fat than this do not work well in baking.

Be careful not to overbake your reduced-fat creations, as they can become dry. Bake cakes and quick breads at 325°F to 350°F, muffins at 350°F, biscuits and scones at 375°F to 400°F, and cookies at 300°F to 325°F. Check the product for doneness a few minutes before the end of the usual baking time. Then enjoy!

Whole Wheat Bread Pudding

Yield: 6 servings

5 slices stale whole wheat bread

⅓ cup dark raisins

½ cup sugar

½ teaspoon ground cinnamon

2 cups skim milk

¼ cup plus 2 tablespoons fat-free egg substitute

1½ teaspoons vanilla extract

1. Cut the bread into ½-inch cubes, and measure the cubes. There should be 5 cups. (Adjust the amount if necessary.)

2. Place the bread cubes in a medium-sized bowl. Add the raisins, and toss to mix. Set aside.

3. Place the sugar and cinnamon in a medium-sized bowl, and stir to mix well. Add the milk, egg substitute, and vanilla extract, and stir to mix well.

4. Pour the milk mixture over the bread cube mixture, and stir gently to mix. Let the mixture sit at room temperature for 10 minutes.

5. Coat a 1½-quart casserole dish with nonstick cooking spray, and pour the bread mixture into the dish. Bake at 350°F for 1 hour, or until a sharp knife inserted in the center of the pudding comes out clean. Let sit for at least 20 minutes before serving. Serve warm or at room temperature, and refrigerate any leftovers.

NUTRITIONAL FACTS (PER ¾-CUP SERVING)

Calories: 178	Fat: 0.9 g	Protein: 8 g
Cholesterol: 1 mg	Fiber: 2.8 g	Sodium: 172 mg

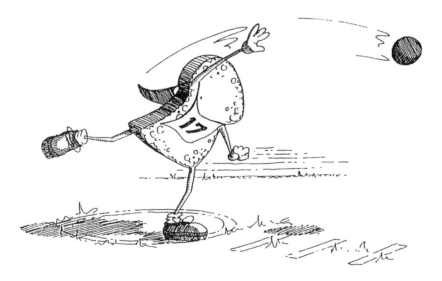

Spiced Cornmeal Pudding

2½-quart pot, and stir to mix well. Slowly stir in the milk and the evaporated milk.

2. Place the pot over medium heat, and cook, stirring constantly, for 10 to 12 minutes, or until the mixture comes to a boil. Reduce the heat to low, and continue to cook and stir for 2 minutes, or until slightly thickened. Slowly stir in the molasses.

3. Place the egg substitute in a small bowl. Remove 1 cup of the hot cornmeal mixture from the pot, and stir it into the egg substitute. Slowly stir the egg mixture into the pudding. Cook and stir for 2 minutes, or until slightly thickened. Remove the pot from the heat, and stir in the vanilla extract and raisins.

4. Coat a 1½-quart round casserole dish with nonstick cooking spray. Pour the pudding mixture into the dish, and place the dish in a pan filled with 1 inch of hot water.

5. Bake uncovered at 350°F for 1 hour and 20 minutes, or until set. When done, a sharp knife inserted midway between the center of the pudding and the rim of the dish should come out clean. Remove the pudding from the oven, and let sit for 30 minutes. Serve warm, or refrigerate for several hours and serve chilled.

¼ cup plus 3 tablespoons whole grain cornmeal

2 tablespoons sugar

½ teaspoon ground cinnamon

½ teaspoon ground ginger

2½ cups skim milk

1 cup evaporated skim milk

⅓ cup molasses

1 cup fat-free egg substitute

1½ teaspoons vanilla extract

⅓ cup dark raisins

NUTRITIONAL FACTS
(PER ⅔-CUP SERVING)

Calories: 157	Fiber: 0.7 g
Chol: 2 mg	Protein: 8.7 g
Fat: 0.4 g	Sodium: 136 mg

FAT-FREE COOKING TIP

Creamy Richness
Without the Cream

To make creamy custards, puddings, and other desserts without the cream, simply replace this high-fat ingredient with an equal amount of evaporated skim milk. Or substitute 1 cup of skim milk plus ⅓ cup of instant nonfat dry milk powder for each cup of cream. Either way, you will save 620 calories and 88 grams of fat for each cup of cream you replace.

Creamy Pineapple Custard

Yield: 7 servings

3 cups skim milk

½ cup instant nonfat dry milk powder

1 cup fat-free egg substitute

½ cup sugar

1 teaspoon vanilla extract

1 can (8 ounces) crushed pineapple in juice, undrained

¼ teaspoon ground nutmeg

1. Place the milk, milk powder, egg substitute, sugar, and vanilla extract in a blender, and blend for 30 seconds to mix well. Stir in the pineapple, including the juice.

2. Coat a 1½-quart baking dish with nonstick cooking spray. Pour the custard mixture into the dish, and sprinkle the top with nutmeg. Place the dish in a pan filled with 1 inch of hot water.

3. Bake uncovered at 350°F for 1 hour and 15 minutes, or until set. When done, a sharp knife inserted midway between the center of the custard and the rim of the dish should come out clean.

4. Remove the dish from the oven, and let cool at room temperature for 1 hour. Cover the dish, and chill for several hours or overnight before serving.

NUTRITIONAL FACTS (PER ¾-CUP SERVING)		
Calories: 146	Fat: 0.2 g	Protein: 9 g
Cholesterol: 3 mg	Fiber: 0.2 g	Sodium: 138 mg

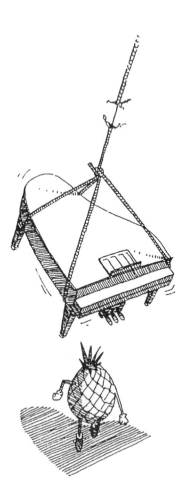

Razzleberry Trifle

medium-sized bowl, and stir to mix well. Set the mixture aside for 20 minutes to let the juices develop.

2. Prepare the pudding with the skim milk according to package directions. Set aside. (If you're using regular pudding, let it chill for 1 to 2 hours before proceeding with the recipe.)

3. Spread one side of each cake slice with a thin layer of the jam. Arrange half of the slices over the bottom of a 3-quart trifle bowl or other decorative glass bowl. Top first with half of the fruit, and then with half of the pudding. Repeat the layers.

4. To make the topping, place the whipped topping in a small bowl, and fold the yogurt into the topping. Swirl the mixture over the top of the trifle, cover, and chill for at least 2 hours before serving.

2½ cups sliced fresh strawberries

1 cup fresh or frozen (thawed) raspberries

2 tablespoons sugar

1 package regular or instant vanilla pudding mix (6-serving size)

3 cups skim milk

10 slices (½-inch each) fat-free loaf cake

¼ cup low-sugar raspberry jam

TOPPING
¾ cup light whipped topping

¾ cup nonfat vanilla yogurt

NUTRITIONAL FACTS (PER 1-CUP SERVING)

Calories: 191	Fat: 1 g	Protein: 5.4 g
Cholesterol: 1 mg	Fiber: 1.5 g	Sodium: 221 mg

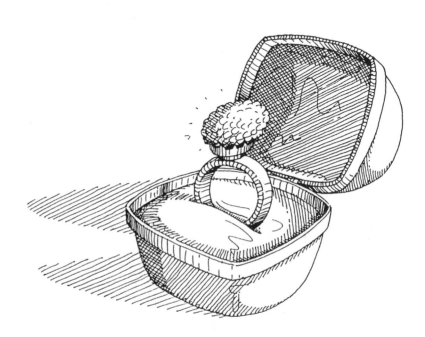

Refreshing Fruit Pie

Yield: 8 servings

CRUST

8 large (2½-x-5-inch) fat-free or reduced-fat graham crackers

3 tablespoons seedless raspberry jam or fruit spread

GLAZE

⅓ cup sugar

3 tablespoons plus 1½ teaspoons cornstarch

1½ cups white grape juice

¼ cup fresh raspberries, slightly crushed

FILLING

3 cups sliced peeled nectarines or peaches (about 3½ medium)

½ cup fresh blueberries

¼ cup fresh raspberries

1. To make the crust, break the crackers into pieces, and place in the bowl of a food processor. Process into fine crumbs. Measure the crumbs. There should be about 1¼ cups. (Adjust the amount if necessary.) Return the crumbs to the food processor, add the jam, and process until the mixture is moist and crumbly.

2. Coat a 9-inch deep dish pie pan with nonstick cooking spray, and use the back of a spoon to press the mixture over the bottom and sides of the pan, forming an even crust. (Periodically dip the spoon in sugar, if necessary, to prevent sticking.) Bake at 350°F for 10 minutes, or until the edges feel firm and dry. Set aside to cool.

3. To make the glaze, place the sugar and cornstarch in a 1-quart saucepan, and stir to mix well. Slowly add the juice, and stir to dissolve the cornstarch. Place the pan over medium heat, and bring to a boil, stirring constantly. Add the raspberries, and cook, still stirring, for another minute, or until the raspberries break up and the glaze turns red. Remove the pan from the heat, and set aside to cool for 15 minutes.

4. Stir the glaze, and spoon a thin layer over the bottom of the crust. Arrange half of the nectarines or peaches in a circular pattern over the crust. Top with the berries, and spoon half of the remaining glaze over the berries. Arrange the rest of the peaches over the glaze, and top with the remaining glaze.

5. Chill for several hours, or until the glaze is set. Cut into wedges and serve cold.

NUTRITIONAL FACTS (PER SERVING)		
Calories: 195	Fat: 0.7 g	Protein: 2.2 g
Cholesterol: 0 mg	Fiber: 2 g	Sodium: 118 mg

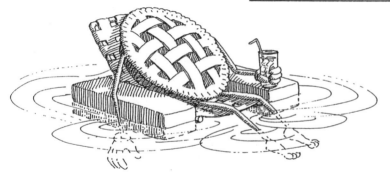

Sweet Potato Pie

1. To make the crust, combine the cereal and sugar in a small bowl, and stir to mix well. Add the egg substitute, and stir to mix well.

2. Coat a 9-inch pie pan with nonstick cooking spray. Use the back of a spoon to press the crust mixture against the bottom and sides of the pan, forming an even crust. Bake at 350°F for 10 minutes, or until the edges feel firm and dry. Set aside to cool.

3. To make the filling, place all of the filling ingredients in a blender or food processor, and process for 1 minute, or until smooth. Pour the filling into the crust. Cut 3-inch wide strips of aluminum foil, and fold over the edges of the pie pan to shield the crust during baking.

4. Bake at 350°F for 50 minutes, or until a sharp knife inserted in the center of the pie comes out clean. Cool to room temperature before cutting into wedges and serving. Refrigerate any leftovers.

Yield: 8 servings

CRUST

1 cup barley nugget cereal

2 tablespoons sugar

3 tablespoons fat-free egg substitute

FILLING

1 can (1 pound) sweet potatoes, drained

1 cup evaporated skim milk

½ cup fat-free egg substitute

½ cup light brown sugar

1½ teaspoons ground cinnamon

½ teaspoon ground nutmeg

1 teaspoon vanilla extract

NUTRITIONAL FACTS (PER SERVING)

Calories: 175	Fat: 0.2 g	Protein: 6.8 g
Cholesterol: 1 mg	Fiber: 2.3 g	Sodium: 175 mg

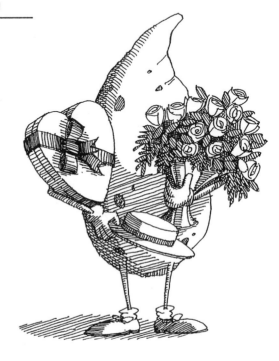

Getting the Fat Out of Your Cookie and Brownie Recipes

As the recipes in this chapter show, a variety of ingredients can be used to replace the fat in cookies and brownies. You can use these same ingredients to get the fat out of your own favorite recipes.

The remainder of this inset will look at the available fat substitutes, and will guide you in using these substitutes to "defat" your cookie and brownie recipes. (For guidelines on modifying muffin, quick bread, and cake recipes, see page 37.) At first, try replacing only half the fat in your recipe. Then try reducing the fat even more. Eventually, your family favorite will be as healthful as it is delicious.

Using Fat Substitutes in Cookies and Brownies

Fat Substitutes	In Which Items Do These Work Best?	How Should Your Recipes Be Modified When Using These Fat Substitutes?
Applesauce, mashed banana, puréed fruits, non-fat buttermilk, and nonfat yogurt.	Use applesauce, buttermilk, or yo-gurt when you want to change the taste as little as possible. Use mashed ba-nanas, puréed rasp-berries, and other fruits for a change of pace.	• Replace part or all of the butter, margarine, or other solid fat in brownies with half as much fat substitute. Replace part or all of the oil with three-fourths as much fat substitute. Mix up the batter, and add more substitute if the batter seems too dry. • Using the same guidelines, replace up to half the fat in cookie recipes. • Replace each whole egg in brownie and cookie recipes with three tablespoons of fat-free egg substitute, if desired. • Bake reduced-fat brownies at 325°F, and check for doneness a few minutes before the end of the usual baking time. Remove the brownies from the oven as soon as the edges are firm and the center is almost set. • Bake reduced-fat cookies at 275°F to 300°F, and bake for 15 to 20 minutes, or until lightly browned.
Honey, maple syrup, molasses, corn syrup, Fruit Source liquid, chocolate syrup, fruit jams and spreads, and fruit juice concentrates.	Use honey or fruit jam in oatmeal cookies; chocolate syrup in brownies; and maple syrup or molasses in spice cookies. Use corn syrup and Fruit Source liquid when you want to change the taste as little as possible. Use fruit juice concentrates in oatmeal and spice cookies.	• Replace part or all of the butter, margarine, or other solid fat in cookies and brownies with three-fourths as much fat substitute. Replace part or all of the oil with an equal amount of fat substitute. Mix up the batter, and add more substitute if the batter seems too dry. Note that totally fat-free cookies will be chewy in texture. If you want crisp cookies, replace no more than half the fat. • Replace each whole egg in cookie recipes with two tablespoons of water. Replace each whole egg in brownie recipes with three tablespoons of fat-free egg substitute, if desired. • Reduce the sugar in cookie and brownie recipes by the amount of fat substitute being added. • Bake reduced-fat brownies at 325°F, and check for doneness a few minutes before the end of the usual baking time. Remove the brownies from the oven as soon as the edges are firm and the center is almost set. • Bake reduced-fat cookies at 275°F to 300°F. Bake for 15 to 20 minutes, or until lightly browned.

Fat Substitutes	In Which Items Do These Work Best?	How Should Your Recipes Be Modified When Using These Fat Substitutes?
160)	licious in brownies and in spice, oatmeal, and chocolate cookies.	brownies and cookies with an equal amount of fat substitute. • Replace each whole egg in brownie and cookie recipes with three tablespoons of fat-free egg substitute, if desired. • Reduce the sugar in cookie and brownie recipes by one-half to two-thirds the amount of fat substitute being used. • Bake reduced-fat brownies at 325°F, and check for doneness a few minutes before the end of the usual baking time. Remove the brownies from the oven as soon as the edges are firm and the center is almost set. • Bake reduced-fat cookies at 350°F, and check for doneness a few minutes before the end of the usual baking time.
Prune Purée (page 160)	Because of Prune Purée's mild flavor, it works well in all recipes.	• Replace part or all of the butter, margarine, or other solid fat in cookies and brownies with half as much Prune Purée. Replace part or all of the oil with three-fourths as much of the purée. • Replace each whole egg in brownie recipes with three tablespoons of egg substitute, if desired. Replace each whole egg in cookie recipes with one egg white or two additional tablespoons of Prune Purée. • Bake reduced-fat brownies at 325°F, and check for doneness a few minutes before the end of the usual baking time. Remove the brownies from the oven as soon as the edges are firm and the center is almost set. • Bake reduced-fat cookies at 350°F, and check for doneness a few minutes before the end of the usual baking time.
Mashed cooked or canned pumpkin, butternut squash, and sweet potatoes	Use any of these substitutes in oatmeal, spice, and chocolate cookie recipes, and in brownies.	• Replace part or all of the butter, margarine, or other solid fat in brownies with one-half to three-fourths as much fat substitute. Replace part or all of the oil with one-half to three-fourths as much fat substitute. Mix up the batter, and add more substitute if the batter seems too dry. • Replace part or all of the butter, margarine, or other solid fat in cookies with one-half to three-fourths as much fat substitute. Replace half of the oil with three-fourths as much fat substitute. Mix up the batter, and add more substitute if the batter seems too dry. • Replace each whole egg in cookie and brownie recipes with three tablespoons of fat-free egg substitute, if desired. • Bake reduced-fat brownies at 325°F, and check for doneness a few minutes before the end of the usual baking time. Remove the brownies from the oven as soon as the edges are firm and the center is almost set. • Bake reduced-fat cookies at 275°F to 300°F, and check for doneness a few minutes before the end of the usual baking time.

Orange Oatmeal Cookies

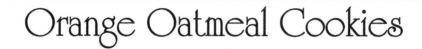

Yield: 42 cookies

1 cup plus 2 tablespoons whole wheat flour

1 cup plus 2 tablespoons quick-cooking oats

⅔ cup sugar

1 teaspoon baking soda

3 tablespoons light corn syrup

2 tablespoons Prune Butter (page 160)

¼ cup plus 2 tablespoons orange juice

½ cup dark raisins or dried cranberries

¼ cup toasted pecans (see inset below)

1. Combine the flour, oats, sugar, and baking soda in a large bowl, and stir to mix well. Add the corn syrup, Prune Butter, and orange juice, and stir to mix well. Fold in the raisins or cranberries and the pecans.

2. Coat a baking sheet with nonstick cooking spray. Drop rounded teaspoonfuls of dough onto the sheet, placing them 1½ inches apart. Slightly flatten each cookie with the tip of a spoon.

3. Bake at 275°F for 18 to 20 minutes, or until golden brown. Cool the cookies on the pan for 1 minute. Then transfer the cookies to wire racks, and cool completely. Serve immediately, or transfer to an airtight container and arrange in single layers separated by sheets of waxed paper.

NUTRITIONAL FACTS (PER COOKIE)

Calories: 48	Fat: 0.6 g	Protein: 0.9 g
Cholesterol: 0 mg	Fiber: 0.8 g	Sodium: 32 mg

LOW-FAT COOKING TIP

Getting the Most Out of Nuts

Nuts add crunch, great taste, and essential nutrients to all kinds of baked goods. Unfortunately, nuts also add fat. But you can halve the fat—without halving the taste—simply by toasting nuts before adding them to your recipe. Toasting intensifies the flavor of nuts so much that you can often cut the amount used in half. Simply arrange the nuts in a single layer on a baking sheet, and bake at 350°F for about 10 minutes, or until lightly browned with a toasted, nutty smell. To save time, toast a large batch and store leftovers in an airtight container in the refrigerator for several weeks, or keep them in the freezer for several months.

and stir to mix well. Add the Prune Purée, honey, and vanilla extract, and stir to mix well. Fold in first the cereal, and then the raisins and the wheat germ or walnuts.

2. Coat a baking sheet with nonstick cooking spray. Drop rounded teaspoonfuls of dough onto the sheet, placing them 1½ inches apart. Slightly flatten each cookie with the tip of a spoon. (Note that the dough will be slightly crumbly, so that you may have to press it together lightly to make it hold its shape.)

3. Bake at 350°F for 8 to 9 minutes, or until lightly browned. Cool the cookies on the pan for 1 minute. Then transfer the cookies to wire racks, and cool completely. Serve immediately, or transfer to an airtight container and arrange in single layers separated by sheets of waxed paper.

1 cup plus 2 tablespoons whole wheat flour

¾ cup sugar

1 teaspoon baking soda

¼ cup plus 2 tablespoons Prune Purée (page 160)

1 tablespoon honey

1 teaspoon vanilla extract

2 cups bran flake cereal

⅓ cup dark raisins

⅓ cup golden raisins

¼ cup toasted wheat germ or chopped walnuts

NUTRITIONAL FACTS (PER COOKIE)

Calories: 44   Fat: 0.2 g   Protein: 1 g
Cholesterol: 0 mg   Fiber: 1 g   Sodium: 44 mg

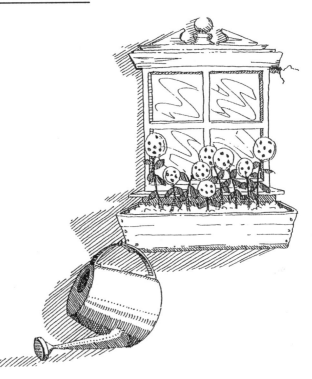

Milk Chocolate Chippers

Yield: 42 cookies

1⅓ cups whole wheat flour

¼ cup instant nonfat dry milk powder

½ cup sugar

¼ cup plus 2 tablespoons brown sugar

¾ teaspoon baking soda

¼ cup plus 2 tablespoons Prune Purée (page 160)

1 teaspoon vanilla extract

½ cup milk chocolate or semi-sweet chocolate chips

⅓ cup dark raisins

¼ cup chopped walnuts (optional)

1. Combine the flour, milk powder, sugars, and baking soda in a large bowl, and stir to mix well. Add the Prune Purée and vanilla extract, and stir to mix well. (The mixture will seem dry at first, but will form a stiff dough as you keep stirring.) Fold in the chocolate chips, the raisins, and, if desired, the walnuts.

2. Coat a baking sheet with nonstick cooking spray. Drop rounded teaspoonfuls of dough onto the sheet, placing them 1½ inches apart. Slightly flatten each cookie with the tip of a spoon.

3. Bake at 350°F for 9 minutes, or until lightly browned. Cool the cookies on the pan for 1 minute. Then transfer the cookies to wire racks, and cool completely. Serve immediately, or transfer to an airtight container and arrange in single layers separated by sheets of waxed paper.

NUTRITIONAL FACTS (PER COOKIE)		
Calories: 43	Fat: 0.7 g	Protein: 0.7 g
Cholesterol: 0 mg	Fiber: 0.7 g	Sodium: 26 mg

Moist and Chewy Brownies

Yield: 16 brownies

¼ cup plus 1 tablespoon unbleached flour

¼ cup oat bran

⅓ cup cocoa powder

¾ cup sugar

¼ cup instant nonfat dry milk powder

1 pinch baking soda

¼ cup chocolate syrup

3 egg whites

1 teaspoon vanilla extract

⅓ cup chopped walnuts (optional)

1. Combine the flour, oat bran, cocoa, sugar, milk powder, and baking soda in a large bowl, and stir to mix well. Stir in the chocolate syrup, egg whites, and vanilla extract. Fold in the nuts if desired.

2. Coat an 8-inch square pan with nonstick cooking spray. Spread the batter evenly in the pan, and bake at 325°F for 23 minutes, or just until the edges are firm and the center is almost set.

3. Cool to room temperature, cut into squares, and serve.

NUTRITIONAL FACTS (PER SERVING)		
Calories: 71	Fat: 0.4 g	Protein: 2 g
Cholesterol: 0 mg	Fiber: 1 g	Sodium: 28 mg

1 ¼ cups whole wheat flour

½ cup oat bran

½ cup plus 2 tablespoons sugar

¼ cup cocoa powder

¾ teaspoon baking soda

¼ cup plus 2 tablespoons Prune Butter (page 160)

¼ cup plus 2 tablespoons chocolate syrup

1 egg white

1 teaspoon vanilla extract

36 pecan halves (optional)

1. Combine the flour, oat bran, sugar, cocoa, and baking soda in a large bowl, and stir to mix well. Add the Prune Butter, chocolate syrup, egg white, and vanilla extract, and stir to mix well. (The mixture will seem dry at first, but will form a stiff dough as you keep stirring.)

2. Coat a baking sheet with nonstick cooking spray. Roll the dough into 1-inch balls, and place 1½ inches apart on the sheet. (If the dough is too sticky to handle, place it in the freezer for a few minutes.) Using the bottom of a glass dipped in sugar, flatten the cookies to ¼-inch thickness. As an alternative, press a pecan half in the center of each cookie to flatten the dough.

3. Bake at 325°F for 10 minutes, or until lightly browned. Cool the cookies on the pan for one minute. Then transfer the cookies to wire racks, and cool completely. Serve immediately, or transfer to an airtight container and arrange in single layers separated by sheets of waxed paper.

NUTRITIONAL FACTS (PER COOKIE)

Calories: 44	Fat: 0.2 g	Protein: 1 g
Cholesterol: 0 mg	Fiber: 1.2 g	Sodium: 30 mg

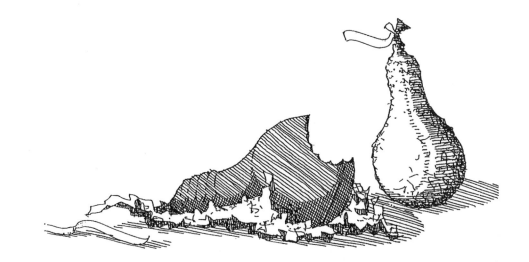

Lemon Meringue Pie

Yield: 8 servings

CRUST

8 large (2½-x-5-inch) fat-free or
reduced-fat graham crackers

2 tablespoons sugar

2 tablespoons fat-free egg substitute

FILLING

¼ cup plus 3 tablespoons cornstarch

¾ cup sugar

1 cup water

¾ cup skim milk

½ cup fat-free egg substitute

¼ cup plus 2 tablespoons lemon juice

1 tablespoon freshly grated lemon rind

MERINGUE TOPPING

3 egg whites, brought to room
temperature

¼ teaspoon cream of tartar

⅛ teaspoon salt

¼ cup plus 1 tablespoon sugar

1 teaspoon vanilla extract

NUTRITIONAL FACTS
(PER SERVING)

Calories: 234   Fiber: 0.6 g
Chol: 0 mg   Protein: 4.2 g
Fat: 0.3 g   Sodium: 199 mg

---

1. To make the crust, break the crackers into pieces, and place in the bowl of a food processor. Process into fine crumbs. Measure the crumbs. There should be about 1¼ cups. (Adjust the amount if necessary.) Return the crumbs to the food processor, add the sugar, and process for a few seconds to mix. Add the egg substitute, and process until the mixture is moist and crumbly.

2. Coat a 9-inch deep dish pie pan with nonstick cooking spray, and use the back of a spoon to press the mixture over the bottom and sides of the pan, forming an even crust. (Periodically dip the spoon in sugar, if necessary, to prevent sticking.) Bake at 350°F for 10 minutes, or until the edges feel firm and dry. Set aside to cool.

3. To make the filling, combine the cornstarch and sugar in a 2-quart saucepan. Slowly stir in the water and milk, and place over medium heat. Cook, stirring constantly with a wire whisk, until the mixture is thickened and bubbly. Reduce the heat to low.

4. Place the egg substitute in a small bowl. Remove ½ cup of the hot filling from the pot, and stir into the egg substitute. Return the mixture to the pot, and cook, stirring constantly, for 2 to 3 minutes, or until the mixture thickens slightly.

5. Remove the pot from the heat, and stir in the lemon juice and rind. Pour the filling into the pie crust, and set aside.

6. To make the meringue, place the egg whites in the bowl of an electric mixer, and beat until foamy. Beat in the cream of tartar and salt, and continue beating until soft peaks form when the beaters are removed. Slowly beat in the sugar, adding 1 tablespoon at a time. Add the vanilla extract, and beat until the mixture is glossy, and stiff peaks form when beaters are removed.

7. Spread the meringue over the warm filling, swirling it with a knife or spoon. Make sure the meringue touches all edges of the crust. Bake at 350°F for about 10 minutes, or just until the meringue is touched with brown.

8. Chill for at least 6 hours before cutting into wedges and serving. For easier serving, dip the knife in warm water before cutting each slice.

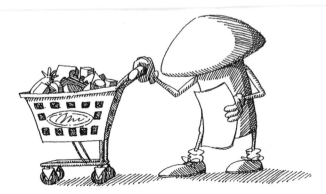

Most of the ingredients used in the recipes in this book are readily available in any supermarket, or can be found in your local health foods or gourmet store. But if you are unable to locate what you're looking for, the following list should guide you to a manufacturer who can either sell the desired product to you directly or inform you of the nearest retail outlet.

Meat Substitutes

Harvest Direct, Inc.
PO Box 4514
Decatur, IL 62525-4514
(800) 835-2867

Harvest Burger mixes, and texturized vegetable protein (TVP).

Nondairy Cheeses

Sharon's Finest
PO Box 5020
Santa Rosa, CA 95402
(800) 656-9669

Almondrella Cheese, Tofurella Cheese, and Veganrella Cheese.

Sweeteners

Fruit Source
1803 Mission Street, Suite 401
Santa Cruz, CA 95060
(408) 457-1136

Fruit Source granulated and liquid sweeteners.

Lundberg Family Farms
PO Box 369
Richvale, CA 95974-0369
(916) 882-4551

Brown rice syrup.

NutraCane, Inc.
5 Meadowbrook Parkway
Milford, NH 03055
(603) 672-2801

Sucanat granulated sweetener.

Vermont Country Maple, Inc.
PO Box 53
Jericho Center, VT 05465
(800) 528-7021

Maple sugar, maple syrup, and other maple products.

Westbrae Natural Foods
1065 East Walnut
Carson, CA 90746
(310) 886-8200

Brown rice syrup and other natural foods.

Whole Grains and Flours

Arrowhead Mills, Inc.
Box 2059
Hereford, TX 79045
(800) 749-0730

Whole wheat pastry flour, oat flour, and other flours and whole grains.

King Arthur Flour
PO Box 876
Norwich, VT 05055
(800) 827-6836

White whole wheat flour and other flours, whole grains, and baking products.

Mountain Ark Trading Company
PO Box 3170
Fayetteville, AR 72702
(800) 643-8909

Whole grains and flours, unrefined sweeteners, dried fruits, fruit spreads, and a wide variety of other natural foods.

Walnut Acres
Walnut Acres Road
Penns Creek, PA 17862
(800) 433-3998
(717) 837-0601

Baking and cooking aids, whole grains and flours, unrefined sweeteners, dried fruits, and a wide variety of other natural foods.

Index

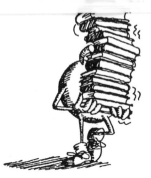